Handbook of Oral Anticoagulation

Handbook of Oral Anticoagulation

Professor Gregory YH Lip
Dr Eduard Shantsila

With contributions from
Dr Deirdre A Lane
Dr Chee W Khoo
Dr Kok Hoon Tay
Dr Suresh Krishnamoorthy

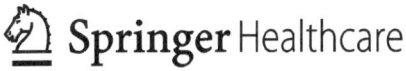 Springer Healthcare

Published by Springer Healthcare, 236 Gray's Inn Road, London, WC1X 8HL, UK

www.springerhealthcare.com

©2010 Springer Healthcare Ltd, a part of Springer Science+Business Media

British Library Cataloguing-in-Publication Data.

A catalogue record for this book is available from the British Library.

ISBN: 978 1 85873 452 1

Although every effort has been made to ensure that drug doses and other information are presented accurately in this publication, the ultimate responsibility rests with the prescribing physician. Neither the publisher nor the authors can be held responsible for errors or for any consequences arising from the use of the information contained herein. Any product mentioned in this publication should be used in accordance with the prescribing information prepared by the manufacturers. No claims or endorsements are made for any drug or compound at present under clinical investigation.

Project editor: Hannah Cole
Designers: Joe Harvey and Taymoor Fouladi
Production: Marina Maher

Contents

Author biographies

Professor Gregory YH Lip is Professor of Cardiovascular Medicine at the University of Birmingham, and Visiting Professor of Haemostasis, Thrombosis and Vascular Sciences in the School of Life and Health Sciences at the University of Aston in Birmingham, UK.

Professor Lip is a member of the scientific documents committee of the European Heart Rhythm Association (EHRA), and serves on the board of the Working Group on Hypertension of the Heart of the European Society of Cardiology (ESC). He is also a member of the Working Groups of Thrombosis and Cardiovascular Pharmacology of the ESC.

Professor Lip has acted as Clinical Adviser for the UK National Institute for Health and Clinical Excellence (NICE) guidelines on atrial fibrillation (AF) management. He was on the writing committee for the 8th American College of Chest Physicians (ACCP) Antithrombotic Therapy Guidelines for Atrial Fibrillation, as well as various guidelines and/or position statements from the EHRA, including the EHRA statement on defining endpoints for AF management, EHRA guidelines for antithrombotic therapy during ablation. He is also on the writing committee for the 2010 ESC Guidelines on Atrial Fibrillation and will be Deputy Editor for the 9th ACCP guidelines on antithrombotic therapy for AF.

Professor Lip is involved at senior editorial level in major international journals, including *Journal of Human Hypertension* (Editor in Chief), *Thrombosis & Haemostasis* (Editor in Chief [Clinical Studies] designate), *Thrombosis Research* (Associate Editor), Europace (Associate Editor) and *Circulation* (Guest Editor). He has published and lectured extensively on thrombosis and antithrombotic disease in cardiovascular disease.

Dr Eduard Shantsila is a Postdoctorate Research Fellow at the University of Birmingham Centre for Cardiovascular Science, City Hospital, Birmingham, UK, where he leads a research group working on a number of research projects that investigate endothelial damage/recovery, and monocyte characteristics including their role in thrombosis in patients with acute coronary syndromes, heart failure, and systemic atherosclerosis.

Dr Shantsila worked in the Republican Research and Practical Centre 'Cardiology', Minsk, Belarus, as a researcher and a cardiologist from 1998 and completed his MD thesis in 2002. From 2005 to 2008 he was a head of the Department of Urgent Cardiology in this centre, where he was actively involved in research work on the problems of cardiovascular diagnostics, endothelial dysfunction and thrombosis.

He is a member of the Working Group of Thrombosis of the European Society of Cardiology.

Dr Shantsila has published extensively on these topics, and is a peer reviewer of major journals in thrombosis.

Dr Deirdre A Lane is a Non-Clinical Lecturer in Medicine at the University of Birmingham Centre for Cardiovascular Sciences, City Hospital, Birmingham, UK. She received her Bachelor of Science with honours from the University of Liverpool in 1995 and her PhD from the University of Birmingham in 2000.

Dr Lane's main research interest is AF, particularly how it affects quality of life and psychological well-being, patient perceptions of the condition, and improving stroke risk and bleeding risk stratification. She is currently the principal investigator on a randomised controlled trial (TREAT- ISCRTN93952605) comparing intensive education with usual care in AF patients newly referred for oral anticoagulation, to examine the impact of education on patients' knowledge and perceptions of AF and its treatment, and INR (international normalised ratio) control. In addition, she is involved in refining the risk stratification of patients requiring oral anticoagulation based on their bleeding risk, in addition to their stroke risk profile. She is the local study coordinator for trials of novel anticoagulants in AF patients.

Dr Lane's background is in health psychology and cardiovascular epidemiology and her other research interests include hypertension, heart failure, cardiac rehabilitation and ethnic differences in cardiovascular disease. She has provided teaching for the European Society of Cardiology Educational Training Programme and is an Associate Editor for Archives in Medical Science.

Dr Lane has published her work widely in journals such as *Stroke*, *Chest*, *Thrombosis and Haemostasis*, *Psychosomatic Medicine*, *Journal of Psychosomatic Research* and *Heart*.

Drs Chee W Khoo, Kok Hoon Tay and Suresh Krishnamoorthy are clinical research fellows in cardiology with interests into the epidemiology and pathophysiology of thromboembolism – and the use of antithrombotic therapy – in cardiovascular disease.

Chapter 1

The coagulation pathway and approaches to anticoagulation

A brief overview of the coagulation pathway

Kok Hoon Tay, Eduard Shantsila, Gregory YH Lip

Intact endothelium is smooth, lacks thrombogenic proteins on its surface and protects circulating blood from exposure to subendothelial proteins such as collagen. As a result, blood constituents flow freely without adhering to endothelial structures. However, when endothelium is damaged and its integrity is disrupted, subendothelial structures come into contact with the constituents of blood (including coagulation factors and platelets), and this triggers an intricate process responsible for platelet attraction and deposition and, simultaneously, the coagulation cascade.

The coagulation cascade comprises two principal elements:

- the tissue factor (extrinsic) pathway
- the contact activation (intrinsic) pathway.

Both pathways ultimately lead to the formation of an insoluble fibrin clot. Each involves a series of reactions in which inactive enzyme precursors are transformed into their active forms, which catalyse the subsequent reactions of the cascade.

The fundamental role of the coagulation system is to facilitate haemostasis when there is haemorrhage due to blood vessel injury. Physiologically, a self-maintained balance of procoagulant and anticoagulant factors/regulators provides a negative feedback system for the prevention of excessive coagulation or haemorrhagic diathesis.

The coagulation cascade

The tissue factor (extrinsic) pathway [1]

When the coagulation cascade is activated, tissue factor (TF), which is normally located in subendothelial tissue, comes into contact with circulating factor VII and forms an activated complex (TF–VIIa) in the presence of Ca^{2+}

(Figure 1.1). TF–VIIa catalyses the conversion of factor X into factor Xa and, following binding of activated factor Va, initiates formation of the serum protease thrombin. Thrombin is formed from prothrombin via a complex reaction in which factors Xa and Va cleave prothrombin fragments 1 and 2 in the presence of Ca^{2+}. Subsequently, thrombin cleaves fibrinopeptides A and B from fibrinogen, resulting in the formation of insoluble fibrin.

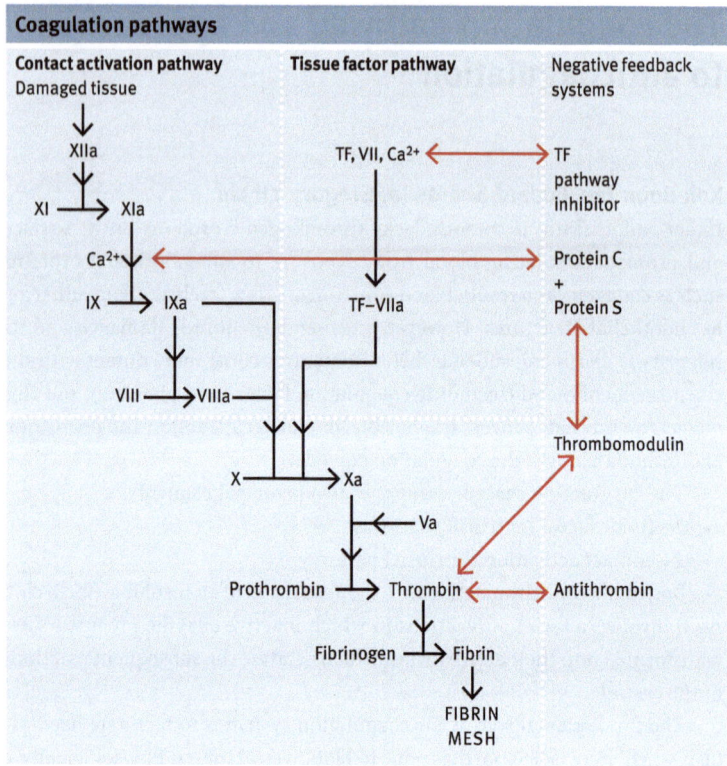

Figure 1.1 Coagulation pathways. TF, tissue factor.

The contact activation (intrinsic) pathway

The contact activation (intrinsic) pathway begins with the formation of a complex made up of Hageman factor (factor XII), prekallikrein, high-molecular-weight kininogen (HMWK) and collagen. Given that the absence of factor XII, prekallikrein or HMWK does not induce a clinically apparent pathology [2], the physiological role of this complex is unclear and it is assumed to have only a minor function in clot formation.

Damage to the endothelial surface triggers formation of factor XIa from factor XI via factor XII. Next, in the presence of Ca^{2+} factor XIa catalyses the conversion of factor IX to IXa, which then triggers the conversion of factor VIII to VIIIa. Factors IXa and VIII form a catalytic complex and efficiently activate factor X. Activation of factor X begins the common pathway, via which the tissue factor and contact activation pathways both result in the formation of a fibrin mesh on the damaged vessel wall.

Regulation of the coagulation cascade

The 'protagonist' of the coagulation cascade is thrombin, which has a master role in regulating the coagulation pathway. Generation of thrombin subsequently activates circulating platelets bound to von Willebrand factor and factor VIIIa.

To avert excessive clotting, multiple elements of a negative feedback system maintain the coagulation cascade in a balanced state. Activated protein C (coupled with protein S) and thrombomodulin limit the excessive generation of factors Va, Xa, VIIIa and IXa. Thus both protein C and protein S act as naturally occurring anticoagulants. Antithrombin, a potent inhibitor of the coagulation cascade, inhibits thrombin and almost all of the clotting factors involved in the cascade. Another mechanism that keeps platelet activation and coagulation under control is mediated by a TF pathway inhibitor, which has its primary role as a restrictor of TF activity.

Conclusions

The coagulation cascade is an intricate process without which haemorrhage/ clotting would occur uncontrollably whenever there is tissue insult.

Approaches to anticoagulation
Eduard Shantsila, Gregory YH Lip

In a large number of disorders there is a raised risk of thrombosis, the pathological development of blood clots that interfere with the circulation. Common examples include:

- venous thromboembolism, encompassing both deep vein thrombosis and pulmonary embolism
- atrial fibrillation
- acute coronary syndromes
- valve disease and endocarditis
- conditions associated with raised risk of ischaemic stroke.

The coagulation cascade is a major target for thromboprophylactic medications. Anticoagulation can be achieved by inhibition of different factors of coagulation. For example, warfarin, discussed in Chapter 3, reduces the functional level of factors II (prothrombin), VII, IX and X by preventing the γ-carboxylation of these vitamin K-dependent factors. However, a disadvantage of warfarin and other vitamin K antagonists is that they are associated with a raised risk of haemorrhage, as described in Chapter 4, together with the fact that their effect fluctuates in any one patient and necessitates frequent monitoring.

Another route exploited for anticoagulation has the use of heparin to increase the inhibitory action of antithrombin. Heparin preparations are the mainstay of anticoagulation in many clinical settings, as reviewed in Chapter 2. However, unlike warfarin, heparin preparations require parenteral administration.

The ideal anticoagulant would be an oral preparation that had more predictable therapeutic action and required significantly less monitoring than warfarin. Consequently, the development of a number of alternative oral anticoagulants is of great interest. Modern novel anticoagulant development has focused on the synthesis of selective plasma factors inhibitors of specific coagulation factors, preferably acting independently of cofactors. The novel oral anticoagulants act on different targets in the coagulation cascade but two key factors, factor Xa and thrombin (factor IIa), appear to be most promising targets, as discussed in Chapter 5. As they are the final elements of the coagulation cascade, their inhibition blocks both the intrinsic (plasma) and the extrinsic (tissue) coagulation cascades.

References

1. Mann KG, Nesheim ME, Church WR, et al. Surface dependent reactions of the vitamin K dependent enzyme complexes. Blood 1990;76:1–16.
2. Badimon L, Badimon JJ. The pathophysiology of thrombus. In: Blann A, Lip GYH, Turpie AGG (eds), Thrombosis in Clinical Practice. London: Taylor & Francis; 2005:1–16.

Chapter 2

Common clinical indications for anticoagulation

Suresh Krishnamoorthy, Chee W Khoo, Eduard Shantsila, Gregory YH Lip

As discussed in Chapter 1, an anticoagulant is a substance that possesses the properties to limit clot formation and therefore can be used therapeutically to prevent or treat thrombotic disorders. In this chapter we discuss the common clinical conditions in which anticoagulation should be considered and the evidence available to justify use of an appropriate antithrombotic therapy in these clinical settings.

Venous thromboembolism

Epidemiology

Venous thromboembolism (VTE) encompasses both deep vein thrombosis (DVT) and pulmonary embolism (PE). It is a common disorder with an incidence of 7.1 per 1,000 person years in developed countries [1,2]. VTE is more common in males and in African-Americans, and the incidence increases with ageing. Furthermore, up to a fifth of patients with previous VTE have recurrences of VTE in the following 5 years [3].

PE, a life-threatening presentation of VTE, has a reported incidence of 2.3 cases per 10,000 person years. Notably, around 80% of cases of PE occur without any clinical signs, two-thirds of lethal outcomes developing within 30 minutes. It is also estimated that 1 in every 100 inpatient deaths is related to PE, making it one of the most common causes of preventable hospital mortality [4].

Given that patients with VTE have a substantially increased risk of morbidity and mortality because of its complications (life-threatening PE and post-thrombotic syndrome) [5], when its presence is suspected patients should be carefully considered to ensure timely diagnosis and initiation of treatment. Common conditions associated with VTE are shown in Figure 2.1. The imbalance between the activated coagulation cascade (both intrinsic and extrinsic pathways) and the fibrinolytic system is another predisposing feature that increases the risk of VTE.

It is worth mentioning that venous thrombi differ in site of formation and are rich in red cells compared with arterial thrombi which are mainly platelet rich. Consequently, the antithrombotic effects of anticoagulants may vary substantially depending on thrombus location and require a specific regimen for clinical setting of venous thrombosis (eg, VTE) and arterial thrombosis (eg, acute coronary syndromes).

Common conditions associated with venous thromboembolism
• Post-trauma
• Post-surgical patients (major surgery lasting > 30 min, orthopaedic surgeries)
• Previous deep vein thrombosis/pulmonary embolism
• Prolonged immobilisation (bed rest, paralysis of legs or plaster casts, long flights)
• Malignancy
• Obesity
• Pregnancy, use of oral contraceptive pills
• Advanced age
• Other conditions: antithrombin III deficiency, protein C and S deficiency (eg, varicose veins, thrombocytosis, polycythaemia rubra vera, systemic lupus erythematosus, nephritic syndrome, stroke and debilitating infections)

Figure 2.1 Common conditions associated with venous thromboembolism.

Anticoagulation in the prevention of venous thromboembolism

The incidence of VTE can be reduced significantly using prophylactic regimens in high-risk patients. Appropriate prophylaxis has been found to be cost effective compared with the cost of managing established VTE cases.

Various prophylactic measures have been recommended in the prevention of VTE, including injections of low-dose unfractionated heparin (UFH), adjusted-dose UFH, low-molecular-weight heparin (LMWH), oral warfarin, external pneumatic compression or gradient elastic stockings alone or in combination. Prophylactic therapy in high-risk patients should be tailored carefully, assessing their individual risk(s) and therapeutic benefits. Nevertheless, in contrast to the management of developed thrombosis, prophylactic therapy is simple, carries minimal risks and, if warfarin is not used, does not require monitoring.

In a meta-analysis of trials (n = 19,958) using parenteral anticoagulant thromboprophylaxis (UFH, LMWH, fondaparinux) in hospitalised medical patients, there was a significant risk reduction in the PE (relative risk [RR] 0.43, 95% confidence interval [CI] 0.26–0.71), fatal PE (RR 0.38, 95% CI 0.21–0.69) and a non-significant reduction in DVT (RR 0.47, 95% CI 0.22–1.00) [6]. Impressively, there was no significant increase in the risk of major haemorrhage (RR 1.32, 95% CI 0.73–2.37) and also no effect on all-cause mortality (RR 0.97, 95% CI 0.790–1.19).

From another meta-analysis of randomised trials [7] ($n = 16,000$), it is clear that compared with placebo perioperative use of prophylactic low-dose UFH reduces the incidence of DVT (odds ratio [OR] 0.3), symptomatic PE (OR 0.5), fatal PE (OR 0.4) and all-cause mortality (OR 0.8) in those undergoing general, orthopaedic and urological surgery. In this analysis, there was also an increase in wound haematomas with low-dose UFH compared with placebo, without any change in the rates of major haemorrhage in these patients [8]. However, the use of UFH was limited due to its shorter half-life and the requirement for repeated injections and monitoring of the activated partial thromboplastin time (APTT).

Because of these limitations, there has been a major switch from low-dose UFH to LMWH (depolymerised UFH). This has both clinical and practical advantages: LMWH has a longer half-life, has higher bioavailability and can be safely administered subcutaneously without the need for monitoring. In one meta-analysis [9], LMWH prophylaxis in patients undergoing general surgery showed a reduction of up to 70% in asymptomatic DVT and symptomatic VTE compared with no prophylaxis. In a meta-analysis assessing the efficacy of individual anticoagulant agents, LMWH appeared to be more effective than UFH in the prevention of asymptomatic DVT (RR 0.47, 95% CI 0.36–0.62), without any increased risk of thrombocytopenia or haemorrhage [10], and it was – unsurprisingly – cost-effective too [11]. Similarly, a meta-analysis of head-to-head trials comparing LMWH and UFH prophylaxis in patients undergoing abdominal, hip and knee surgery showed superior efficacy for LMWH in reducing VTE and deaths related to VTE, with a good safety profile [12–14].

Hopes for further improvement in parenteral management of thrombosis were associated with introduction of the selective factor Xa inhibitor fondaparinux. However, although advantages of fondaparinux were demonstrated in patients with acute coronary syndromes, it has been found to have similar effectiveness and safety to the LMWH dalteparin in patients undergoing high-risk abdominal surgery [15].

Oral anticoagulants for thromboprophylaxis after surgery

Until recently, oral anticoagulants were not considered an option for thromboprophylaxis after surgery. Warfarin could not be recommended for VTE prevention due to its delayed onset of action, its narrow therapeutic range and the requirement for careful monitoring. The novel oral direct thrombin inhibitor ximelagatran achieved optimistic results in initial trials but was removed from further development because of safety issues [16,17]. More recently, however, newer oral anticoagulants have shown promise in thromboprophylaxis after surgery, and trials are continuing (see Chapter 5).

Recommendations from the ACCP evidence-based clinical practice guidelines for the prevention of venous thromboembolism	
Conditions associated with moderate-to-high risk for VTE	Recommendations
General surgery in moderate-to-high risk patients	LDUH or LMWH ± GCS or IPC (grade 1A)
Vascular surgery + thromboembolic risk factors	LDUH or LMWH (grade 1C)
Gynaecological surgery + thromboembolic risk factors	LDUH or LMWH (grade 1A)
Urological surgery (major, open)	LDUH (grade 1A) or LMWH (grade 1C)
Laparoscopic surgery + thromboembolic risk factors	LDUH or LMWH or IPC or GCS (grade 1C)
Elective hip arthroplasty	LMWH or fondaparinux or adjusted-dose VKA (INR 2–3) (all grade 1A)
Elective knee arthroplasty	LMWH or fondaparinux or adjusted-dose VKA (INR 2–3) (all grade 1A)
High-risk neurosurgery	LDUH or LMWH ± GCS or IPC (grade 2B)
Trauma + at least one risk factor for VTE	LMWH (grade 1A)
Spinal cord injuries	LMWH ± IPC (grade 1B) or LDUH (grade 2B)
Burns + risk factors for VTE	LMWH or LDUH (grade 1C)
Medical conditions (CHF, severe respiratory disease, confined to bed or with additional risk factors including active cancer, previous VTE, sepsis, acute neurological disease, inflammatory bowel disease)	LMWH or LDUH (both grade 1A) GCS or IPC, if contraindications to anticoagulation (grade 1C)
Long-distance travel + risk factors for VTE	Below knee GCS (15–30 mm Hg) at the ankles or single dose of LMWH prior to departure (grade 2B)

Figure 2.2 Recommendations from the ACCP evidence-based clinical practice guidelines for the prevention of venous thromboembolism. ACCP, American College of Chest Physicians; CHF, congestive heart failure; GCS, gradient compression stockings; INR, international normalised ratio; IPC, intermittent pneumatic compression; LDUH, low-dose unfractionated heparin; LMWH, low-molecular-weight heparin; VKA, vitamin K antagonist; VTE, venous thromboembolism.

Guidelines for prevention of VTE

The risk of VTE is not homogeneous and depends on the presence of concomitant risk factors. The American College of Chest Physicians (ACCP) have published evidence-based clinical practice guidelines on VTE prevention following surgery and other medical conditions (Figure 2.2) [18].

Treatment of venous thromboembolism

A number of randomised trials have confirmed that in patients with lower-limb DVT, LMWH is superior to UFH in reducing mortality at 3–6 months and reducing the risk of haemorrhage [19]. Furthermore, a meta-analysis of trials comparing UFH and LMWH [20] for the treatment of VTE showed no difference in the recurrence of VTE or PE in minor or major haemorrhage, or in thrombocytopenia. A 24% reduction in total mortality was observed in patients treated with LMWH compared with UFH (RR 0.76, 95% CI 0.59–0.98). Treatment of PE with LMWH also appears to be safe, being at least as effective as UFH, and also cost effective, without the need for special laboratory monitoring [15,21,22].

In the Matisse DVT trial [23], once-daily subcutaneous administration of fondaparinux was found to be non-inferior to twice-daily injection of the LMWH enoxaparin, with no differences in the recurrence of DVT, major haemorrhage or death at 3 months. LMWHs have also proved to be effective and safe options for the outpatient treatment of VTE [24–26].

A disadvantage to LMWHs is that they do require daily subcutaneous injections of the medicine, often by trained personnel. Consequently, oral anticoagulation is considered an attractive option. Available data indicate that warfarin is non-inferior to LMWH in patients with VTE (without cancers), with a similar rate of VTE recurrence or haemorrhage [27]. Of interest, these positive results with warfarin were noted despite patients spending a relatively low proportion of time within the therapeutic international normalised ratio (INR) range, thus mirroring real life primary care practice. However, in patients with coexistent malignancies, treatment with LMWH appears to be more efficacious compared with warfarin [28].

Decisions with regard to the duration of warfarin anticoagulation in patients with VTE should be guided by whether or not the aetiology is idiopathic. In the various trials the VTE patient cohort has been highly heterogeneous; nevertheless, it is clear from the pooled analyses that, compared with early termination of treatment, prolonged anticoagulation with warfarin (INR 2–3) is associated with significant reduction in the recurrence of VTE [29–31], albeit with a non-significant increase in the risk of haemorrhage. Conventional intensive therapy (INR 2–3) has also been found to be more effective than low-intensity (INR 1.5–2) anticoagulation [32,33], without any increased risk of haemorrhage in patients with symptomatic VTE.

The indirect factor Xa inhibitor idraparinux (injected subcutaneously once weekly) was found in a recent randomised trial [34] to be as effective and safe as warfarin in patients with VTE, with no differences in DVT recurrence. However, idraparinux was comparatively less effective in patients with PE, and long-term therapy carried higher haemorrhage risks than did warfarin.

As an alternative to oral and parenteral anticoagulation for VTE management, catheter-directed thrombolysis [35–37] and thrombus removal [38] can be used and have been shown to improve the venous patency and outcomes in patients with acute DVT. In contrast, the available evidence for the utility of inferior vena cava filters [39,40] for treatment of VTE is conflicting, and therefore their routine use is not recommended. If they are used, patients should also receive conventional anticoagulation treatment. With regard to thrombolysis in acute PE, a meta-analysis of trials [41] comparing thrombolysis with heparin has shown a non-significant reduction in PE recurrence (OR 0.67, 95% CI 0.4–1.12) and all-cause mortality (OR 0.70, 95% CI 0.37–1.30) with thrombolysis, but this was achieved at the expense of significantly higher non-major haemorrhage (OR 2.63, 95% CI 1.53–4.54) and intracranial haemorrhages.

Guidelines for treatment of venous thromboembolism

Current guidelines [42,43] recommend long-term oral anticoagulation at a conventional intensity (INR 2–3 for vitamin K antagonist [VKA]) for patients with VTE (Figure 2.3). The duration of the treatment should be 3–6 months in those with precipitating risk factors and 12 months for 'idiopathic' VTE. However, in the event of further recurrences, the therapy should be further extended (for 12 months or more). Thrombolysis in patients with PE is reserved for those with haemodynamic instability or with other poor prognostic features such as hypoxia, dilated and hypokinetic right ventricle, or elevated cardiac markers. Importantly, precipitating factors such as occult malignancies (4–10% of VTE cases) [44] should be carefully considered in VTE patients, particularly in those with 'idiopathic VTE'.

Atrial fibrillation
Epidemiology and thromboembolic risks with AF
The prevalence and incidence of atrial fibrillation (AF) are high and increase with advancing age. The overall prevalence of AF was 6% in the Framingham and Rotterdam studies [45,46]. Both these studies found a one in four lifetime

Recommendations from the ACCP evidence-based clinical practice guidelines for the prevention of venous thromboembolism	
Conditions requiring treatment with anticoagulation	**Recommendations**
Acute DVT	
Initial treatment	LMWH or UFH or fondaparinux (all grade 1A)
Long-term treatment	
With a reversible cause	Adjusted VKA (INR 2–3) for 3 months (grade 1A)
Unprovoked DVT	Adjusted VKA (INR 2–3) for at least 3 months (grade 1A) and long term (grade 1C) reassessing risk-benefit ratio
Second episode of unprovoked DVT	Adjusted VKA (INR 2–3) long term (grade 1A)
Acute PE	
Initial treatment	
With haemodynamic compromise, hypoxia, right heart dilatation or hypokinesis	Thrombolysis
With no haemodynamic compromise	LMWH or UFH or fondaparinux (all grade 1a)
Long term	
PE with reversible risk factor	Adjusted-dose VKA (INR 2–3) for 3 months (grade 1A)
Unprovoked PE	Adjusted-dose VKA (INR 2–3) for at least 3 months (grade 1A) and long term (grade 1C) reassessing risk–benefit ratio
Second episode of VTE	Adjusted-dose VKA (INR 2–3) long term (grade 1A)

Figure 2.3 Recommendations from the ACCP evidence-based clinical practice guidelines for the prevention of venous thromboembolism. DVT, deep vein thrombosis; LMWH, low-molecular-weight heparin; INR, Internationalised normal ratio; PE, pulmonary embolism; UFH, unfractionated heparin; VKA, vitamin K antagonists.

risk of developing AF, for both men and women aged 40 years and above. The population-based Renfrew–Paisley study in west Scotland found the prevalence of AF among patients aged 45–64 years to be 6.5% [47]. The prevalence of AF increases with age and is higher in males. The incidence of AF has risen by 13% over the past two decades, and it is predicted that 15.9 million people in the USA will have AF by 2050 [48].

The clinical significance of AF is largely associated with its increased risk for thromboembolic complications. In fact, the risk of ischaemic stroke or thromboembolism is four- to five-fold higher across all age groups in patients with AF, and is similar in patients with either paroxysmal or permanent AF [49].

Acute AF

At present no clinical trial data are available assessing the role of anticoagulation in acute AF with haemodynamic instability. Consensus statements made by the UK National Institute for Health and Clinical Excellence (NICE) and the AHA/ACC/ESC guidelines (2006) [50] advocate the use of heparin prior to cardioversion in acute AF, irrespective of the method used. In a randomised clinical trial of 155 patients with AF duration between 2 and 19 days and undergoing transoesophageal echocardiography-guided cardioversion, no significant differences between UFH and LMWH were observed in rates of stroke, systemic embolism, thrombus formation or haemorrhage [51]. The use of LMWH simplifies the treatment regimen and allows early discharge from hospital [52]. However, for patients with planned cardioversion (whether electrical or pharmacological), oral anticoagulation has to be initiated and therapeutic levels maintained for at least 3 weeks before and 4 weeks after the procedure.

Long-term oral anticoagulation should be considered in patients with stroke risk factors or if there is a high risk of AF recurrence. If successful cardioversion has not been achieved, the need for long-term thromboprophylaxis should be assessed according to the patient's individual stroke risk.

Independent risk factors for stroke and thromboembolism
1. Prior stroke or transient ischaemic attack
2. Diabetes mellitus
3. Hypertension
4. Older age

Figure 2.4 Independent risk factors for stroke and thromboembolism.

Long-term thromboprophylaxis

The long-term risk of stroke is not homogeneous among AF patients. Each patient with AF should be assessed for thromboembolic risk, contraindications and comorbidities prior to commencement of antithrombotic therapy. In a systematic review, the Stroke in AF Working Group has identified several independent risk factors for stroke and thromboembolism in AF patients, and these are listed in Figure 2.4 [53].

Thromboprophylaxis in atrial fibrillation: clinical trials comparing warfarin with control				
Study	**Number of patients (warfarin)**	**Target INR**	**Thromboembolic event/patients, warfarin vs placebo**	**RRR (%); comments**
AFASAK [75]	671 (335)	2.8–4.2	5/335 vs 21/336	54
BAATAF [76]	420(212)	1.5–2.7	3/212 vs 13/208	78
CAFA [77]	378 (187)	2.0–3.0	6/187 vs 9/191	33
EAFT [78] (secondary prevention study)	439 (225)	2.5–4.0	20/225 vs 50/214	68; mean follow-up 2.3 years; annual rate of outcome event was 8% vs 17%
SPAF-I [79]	421 (210)	2.0–4.5	8/210 vs 19/211	60
SPINAF [80]	571 (281)	1.4–2.8	7/281 vs 23/290	70; mean follow up 1.8 years; annual event rate among patients over 70 years of age: 4.8% in placebo group, 0.9% in warfarin group (risk reduction 0.79)

Figure 2.5 Thromboprophylaxis in atrial fibrillation: clinical trials comparing warfarin with control. AFASAK, Atrial Fibrillation, Aspirin, Anticoagulation trial; BAATAF, Boston Area Anticoagulation Trial for Atrial Fibrillation; CAFA, Canadian Atrial Fibrillation Anticoagulation trial; EAFT, European Atrial Fibrillation Trial; INR, international normalised ratio; RRR, relative risk reduction; SPAF, Stroke Prevention in Atrial Fibrillation trial; SPINAF, Stroke Prevention in Non-rheumatic Atrial Fibrillation trial.

Warfarin versus placebo

The clinical trials that have compared warfarin with either control or placebo are summarised in Figure 2.5. The results of these trials and a meta-analysis of adjusted-dose warfarin [54,55] in AF patients showed a two-thirds reduction, compared with placebo, in the relative risk of ischaemic stroke or systemic embolism in high-risk patients.

Aspirin versus placebo

The clinical trials that have compared antiplatelet therapy with either placebo or control are summarised in Figure 2.6. Various aspirin doses between 50 and 1200 mg/day) have been employed in these trials and

Thromboprophylaxis in atrial fibrillation: clinical trials comparing aspirin with control			
Study	Number of patients (aspirin)	Doses (mg/day)	Thromboembolic event/ patients, RRR (%); comments
AFASAK [56]	672 (336)	75	16/336 vs 19/336; 17
EAFT [59]	782 (404)	300	88/404 vs 90/378; 11
ESPS Π [81]	211 (104)	50	17/104 vs 23/107, at mean follow-up of 2 years. Stroke risk was reduced by 18% with aspirin compared with placebo.
SPAF 1 [60]	1120 (552)	325	25/552 vs 44/568; 44
UK-TIA [82]	(a) 28 (13) (b) 36 (21)	300 1200	(a) 3/13 vs 4/15; 17 (b) 5/21 vs 4/15; 14
JAST [83]	871 (426)	150	20/426 vs 19/445; 10
LASAF [84]	(a) 195 (104) (b) 181 (90)	125 125 mg/alt day	(a) 4/104 vs 3/91; 17 (b) 1/90 vs 3/91; 67

Figure 2.6 Thromboprophylaxis in atrial fibrillation: clinical trials comparing aspirin with control. AFASAK, Atrial Fibrillation, Aspirin, Anticoagulation trial; alt, alternate; EAFT, European Atrial Fibrillation Trial; ESPS, European Stroke Prevention Study; JAST, Japan Atrial Fibrillation Stroke Trial; LASAF, Low-dose Aspirin, Stroke, Atrial Fibrillation; RRR, relative risk reduction; SPAF, Stroke Prevention in Atrial Fibrillation trial; UK-TIA, United Kingdom Transient Ischaemic Attack.

evaluated during follow-up periods ranging from 1.2 years to 4.0 years. Recent meta-analyses [54,56] have reported that antiplatelet drugs, when compared with controls, reduced overall stroke risk by 19–22%. However, this magnitude of stroke reduction is similar to that seen by the use of antiplatelet therapy in high-risk vascular disorders and, given that AF commonly coexists with vascular disease, the effect of aspirin may simply reflect the effect on vascular disease.

Warfarin versus antiplatelet therapy

A meta-analysis of 12 large randomised trials [54] involving 12,721 participants found a 39% RR reduction in all strokes when INR-adjusted-dose warfarin was compared with aspirin. The Clopidogrel plus aspirin versus oral anticoagulation for AF in the Atrial fibrillation Clopidogrel Trial with Irbesartan for prevention of Vascular Events (ACTIVE-W) [57], the largest of these trials, was stopped early because of the clear evidence of superiority of adjusted-dose warfarin.

In the recent randomised Birmingham Atrial Fibrillation Treatment of the Aged (BAFTA) study [58], warfarin (INR 2–3) was compared with aspirin 75 mg/day in 973 patients with AF aged 75 years or older in a primary care setting. The study demonstrated that during the average 2.7-year follow-up warfarin was significantly more effective than aspirin in preventing stroke (by over 50%, with nearly 2% annual absolute risk reduction), without any difference between warfarin and aspirin in the risk of major haemorrhage.

At present, adjusted-dose warfarin remains the most efficacious prophylaxis for AF patients who have at least moderate risk of stroke.

Anticoagulation in other medical conditions

Valve disease and endocarditis

In patients with prosthetic mechanical heart valves, oral anticoagulation offers superior and consistent protection against systemic thromboembolism compared with antiplatelet agents and is therefore recommended in all such patients [59]. According to current consensus recommendations, mechanical prosthetic valves at the aortic position require an INR of 2.0–3.0, whereas valves at the mitral position require an INR of 2.5–3.5 for the satisfactory prevention of thrombus formation. However, mechanical prosthetic mitral 'ball-cage' valve prosthesis may require even higher INR levels (4.0–4.9) for adequate thromboprophylaxis and, consequently, need tight laboratory monitoring.

Oral anticoagulation is also recommended in patients with bioprosthetic valves in both the mitral and the aortic position, to minimise acute thromboembolic risk. The recommended duration of anticoagulation for this indication is 3 months after prosthesis implantation, although the evidence supporting its efficacy is not compelling, and the risk of haemorrhage appears to be increased even with INR ranges of 2.0–3.0.

Both infective and non-bacterial thrombotic endocarditis carry a higher risk of embolic stroke. Persistent vegetation of >10 mm despite treatment, or one or more embolic events in the first 2 weeks of treatment, are indications for acute surgical treatment of the affected valves [60]. Nevertheless data on the benefits of anticoagulant drugs in these clinical settings are lacking.

Acute myocardial infarction, left ventricular thrombus and aneurysm

The risk of stroke associated with acute myocardial infarction (MI) accompanied by left ventricular (LV) mural thrombus can be as high as 15% [61]. Nearly half of all patients with LV aneurysm have LV thrombus, and in such patients the extent of MI, severity of LV dysfunction and age are independent predictors of stroke [62]. Anticoagulation has been associated with a 68% risk reduction in stroke in post-MI patients with LV thrombus and is now recommended for 3 months where LV thrombus formation post-MI occurs [63].

Trials evaluating effectiveness of oral anticoagulation in post-MI patients have shown conflicting and inconclusive results. In a subgroup of patients with AF post-MI in the Efficacy and Safety of the oral direct Thrombin inhibitor ximElagatran in patients with rEcent Myocardial damage (ESTEEM) trial, the combination of ximelagatran and aspirin (6.9%) significantly reduced the risk of death, non-fatal MI and stroke (20.6%) during a 6-month follow-up, compared with aspirin alone [64]. The Coumadin Aspirin Reinfarction study (CARS) [65] compared fixed low-dose warfarin (INR 1.3–1.8) with low-dose aspirin (80 mg) and found no difference in the non-fatal reinfarction or non-fatal stroke or cardiovascular death (8.6% with aspirin vs. 8.4% with warfarin) at a median of 14 months of follow-up. Similar results were obtained in the Combination Haemotherapy and Mortality Prevention (CHAMP) trial [66]; this compared aspirin monotherapy with warfarin (mean INR 1.8) plus aspirin after acute MI, and found no differences in stroke (3.5% with aspirin and 3.1% with combination therapy) at a median 2.7-year follow-up.

In contrast, the Warfarin, Aspirin, Reinfarction (WARIS) II study [67] showed that anticoagulation with warfarin plus aspirin or with warfarin alone (within 4 weeks of MI) reduced mortality, non-fatal reinfarction or stroke compared with aspirin alone (15% vs 16.7% vs. 20%, respectively). There was an overall risk reduction of 29% with combination therapy and 19% with warfarin at a median follow-up of 2.7 years, but at the expense of more haemorrhagic events in the warfarin groups compared with aspirin alone (0.62% vs 0.17% per treatment year). The Antithrombotics in the Secondary Prevention of Events in Coronary Thrombosis-2 (ASPECT-2) study [68] showed similar benefits of oral anticoagulation compared with antiplatelet therapy; there was a reduction in mortality, MI and strokes (9% aspirin vs 5% warfarin vs 5% warfarin plus aspirin), but with a trend towards higher haemorrhage rate with warfarin.

Nonetheless, there is still no clear consensus as to whether anticoagulant treatment of the whole cohort of patients with acute MI in sinus rhythm is more effective compared with conventional treatment with antiplatelets in reducing adverse cardiac events and, if it is, how long the treatment should continue.

In patients with coronary artery disease who require percutaneous intervention but are anticoagulated because of concomitant disorders such as AF, VTE or prosthetic heart valves, current recommendations suggest the use of bare metal stents and short-term triple therapy of aspirin, clopidogrel and warfarin to avoid recurrent cardiac ischaemia and/or stent thrombosis, and thereafter changing to warfarin plus clopidogrel to minimise haemorrhage risks [69].

Heart failure

Heart failure is an increasingly common condition, and is associated with increased thromboembolic risk. However, the utility of chronic anticoagulant therapy in patients with heart failure is still controversial. The authors of a Cochrane systematic review of antithrombotic drugs in patients with heart failure found no robust evidence for additional benefits of anticoagulation over administration of aspirin in reducing mortality and thromboembolism. Of note, hospitalisations were more common in aspirin users than in those managed with warfarin [70,71].

Possible benefits of long-term oral anticoagulation have been addressed in several recent trials (Figure 2.7). For example, the Warfarin/Aspirin Study in Heart Failure (WASH) trial was a small pilot study [72] that compared aspirin, warfarin and no treatment in heart failure patients. It found no statistical differences in the primary endpoints of death, non-fatal MI or non-fatal stroke (26, 32 and 26%, respectively), after a mean follow up of 27 months. Nonetheless, the rate of hospitalisation was significantly higher in the aspirin arm compared with the warfarin arm and the no-treatment arm.

Heart failure: summary of randomised clinical trials comparing warfarin and aspirin			
Trials	Follow-up (in months)	Head-to-head comparison	Results
WASH	27	Warfarin ($n = 89$) vs aspirin ($n = 91$) vs no treatment ($n = 99$)	No differences observed in primary outcomes (death or non-fatal MI or stroke) between treatment groups. More patients in aspirin group than warfarin group had CV-related hospitalisations or death (HR 1.39, 95%CI 0.95–2.00) during first 12 months of follow-up.
WATCH	18	Warfarin ($n = 540$) vs aspirin ($n = 523$) or clopidogrel ($n = 524$)	No significant differences noted in primary outcomes (death or non-fatal MI or non-fatal strokes) between treatment groups. However, patients on aspirin had more heart failure related hospitalisations than those on warfarin ($p = 0.019$)

Figure 2.7 Heart failure: summary of randomised clinical trials comparing warfarin and aspirin. CI, confidence interval; CV, cardiovascular; HR, hazard ratio; MI, myocardial infarction; WASH,

Similar results were seen in the Warfarin and Antiplatelet Therapy in Chronic Heart failure (WATCH) trial [73], in which patients with ejection fraction <35% were randomised to blinded antiplatelet therapy (aspirin or clopidogrel) or warfarin to prevent thromboembolic events. In this study no difference was observed in the primary endpoints of stroke, MI or death (20.5 vs 21 vs 19.8%, respectively) at 18 months follow-up. However, because of poor recruitment of patients, the study was terminated earlier than expected and therefore was underpowered.

The ongoing multicentre, double-blind, randomised Warfarin versus Aspirin with Reduced Ejection Fraction (WARCEF) trial [74] is studying the benefits of warfarin or aspirin in heart failure patients and may provide evidence for the benefits of appropriate antithrombotic therapy in these patients.

Conclusions

Compelling evidence favours use of appropriate antithrombotic therapies for the prevention of VTE as well as treatment of patients with VTE, AF and implantation of prosthetic valves, and the range of indications for anticoagulant therapy may expand further. However, despite this, each patient who might require anticoagulation should be individually assessed in terms of the potential benefits and risks of the therapy. Furthermore, the approach towards treatment needs to be holistic, and success is largely based on appropriate patient education to facilitate safer and effective use of anticoagulant therapies.

References

1. Heit JA, Melton LJ 3rd, Lohse CM, et al. Incidence of venous thromboembolism in hospitalized patients vs community residents. Mayo Clin Proc 2001;76:1102–10.
2. Fowkes FJ, Price JF, Fowkes FG. Incidence of diagnosed deep vein thrombosis in the general population: systematic review. Eur J Vasc Endovasc Surg 2003;25:1–5.
3. Hansson PO, Sörbo J, Eriksson H. Recurrent venous thromboembolism after deep vein thrombosis: incidence and risk factors. Arch Intern Med 2000;160:769–74.
4. Morrell MT, Dunnill MS. The post-mortem incidence of pulmonary embolism in a hospital population. Br J Surg 1968;55:347–52.
5. Heit JA, Silverstein MD, Mohr DN, et al. Predictors of survival after deep vein thrombosis and pulmonary embolism: a population-based, cohort study. Arch Intern Med 1999;159:445–53.
6. Dentali F, Douketis JD, Gianni M, et al. Meta-analysis: anticoagulant prophylaxis to prevent symptomatic venous thromboembolism in hospitalized medical patients. Ann Intern Med 2007;146:278–88.
7. Collins R, Scrimgeour A, Yusuf S, Peto R. Reduction in fatal pulmonary embolism and venous thrombosis by perioperative administration of subcutaneous heparin. Overview of results of randomized trials in general, orthopedic, and urologic surgery. N Engl J Med 1988;318:1162–73.
8. Clagett GP, Reisch JS. Prevention of venous thromboembolism in general surgical patients: results of meta-analysis. Ann Surg 1988;208:227–40.
9. Mismetti P, Laporte S, Darmon JY, et al. Meta-analysis of low molecular weight heparin in the prevention of venous thromboembolism in general surgery. Br J Surg 2001;88,913–30.
10. Wein L, Wein S, Haas SJ, et al. Pharmacological venous thromboembolism prophylaxis in hospitalized medical patients: a meta-analysis of randomized controlled trials. Arch Intern Med 2007;167:1476–86.
11. Deitelzweig SB, Becker R, Lin J, Benner J. Comparison of the two-year outcomes and costs of prophylaxis in medical patients at risk of venous thromboembolism. Thromb Haemost 2008;100:810–20.
12. Nurmohamed MT, Rosendaal FR, Büller HR, et al. Low-molecular-weight heparin versus standard heparin in general and orthopaedic surgery: a meta-analysis. Lancet 1992;340:152–6.
13. Hull RD, Raskob GE, Pineo G, et al. A comparison of subcutaneous low-molecular-weight heparin with warfarin sodium for prophylaxis against deep-vein thrombosis after hip or knee implantation. N Engl J Med 1993;329:1370–6.
14. Francis CW, Pellegrini VD Jr, Totterman S, et al. Prevention of deep-vein thrombosis after total hip arthroplasty. Comparison of warfarin and dalteparin. J Bone Joint Surg Am 1997;79:1365–72.
15. Agnelli, G, Bergqvist, D, Cohen, A, et al. Randomized double-blind study to compare the efficacy and safety of postoperative fondaparinux (Arixtra) and preoperative dalteparin in the prevention of venous thromboembolism after high-risk abdominal surgery: the PEGASUS Study [abstract]. Blood 2003;102,15a.

16. Francis CW, Berkowitz SD, Comp PC, et al.; EXULT A Study Group. Comparison of ximelagatran with warfarin for the prevention of venous thromboembolism after total knee replacement. N Engl J Med 2003;349:1703–12.

17. Colwell CW Jr, Berkowitz SD, Lieberman JR, et al.; EXULT B Study Group. Oral direct thrombin inhibitor ximelagatran compared with warfarin for the prevention of venous thromboembolism after total knee arthroplasty. J Bone Joint Surg Am 2005;87:2169–77.

18. Geerts WH, Bergqvist D, Pineo GF, et al. American College of Chest Physicians. Prevention of venous thromboembolism: American College of Chest Physicians Evidence-Based Clinical Practice Guidelines (8th Edition). Chest 2008;133:381–453S.

19. Howard PA. Dalteparin: a low-molecular-weight heparin. Ann Pharmacother 1997;31:92–203.

20. Dolovich LR, Ginsberg JS, Douketis JD, et al. A meta-analysis comparing low-molecular-weight heparins with unfractionated heparin in the treatment of venous thromboembolism: examining some unanswered questions regarding location of treatment, product type, and dosing frequency. Arch Intern Med 2000;160:181–8.

21. Green D, Hirsh J, Heit J, et al. Low molecular weight heparin: a critical analysis of clinical trials. Pharmacol Rev 1994;46:89–109.

22. Raschke R, Hirsh J, Guidry JR. Suboptimal monitoring and dosing of unfractionated heparin in comparative studies with low-molecular-weight heparin. Ann Intern Med 2003;138:720–3.

23. Büller HR, Davidson BL, Decousus H, et al.; Matisse Investigators. Fondaparinux or enoxaparin for the initial treatment of symptomatic deep venous thrombosis: a randomized trial. Ann Intern Med 2004;140:867–73.

24. Vinson DR, Berman DA. Outpatient treatment of deep venous thrombosis: a clinical care pathway managed by the emergency department. Ann Emerg Med 2001;37:251–8.

25. Smith BJ, Weekley JS, Pilotto L, et al. Cost comparison of at-home treatment of deep venous thrombosis with low molecular weight heparin to inpatient treatment with unfractionated heparin. Intern Med J 2002;32:29–34.

26. Segal JB, Streiff MB, Hofmann LV, et al. Management of venous thromboembolism: a systematic review for a practice guideline. Ann Intern Med 2007;146:211–22.

27. Das SK, Cohen AT, Edmondson RA, et al. Low-molecular-weight heparin versus warfarin for prevention of recurrent venous thromboembolism: a randomized trial. World J Surg 1996;20:521–6.

28. Lee AY, Levine MN, Baker RI, et al.; Randomized Comparison of Low-Molecular-Weight Heparin versus Oral Anticoagulant Therapy for the Prevention of Recurrent Venous Thromboembolism in Patients with Cancer (CLOT) Investigators. Low-molecular-weight heparin versus a coumarin for the prevention of recurrent venous thromboembolism in patients with cancer. N Engl J Med 2003;349:146–53.

29. Agnelli G, Prandoni P, Santamaria MG, et al.; Warfarin Optimal Duration Italian Trial Investigators. Three months versus one year of oral anticoagulant therapy for idiopathic deep venous thrombosis. Warfarin Optimal Duration Italian Trial Investigators. N Engl J Med 2001;345:165–9.

30. Schulman S, Rhedin AS, Lindmarker P, et al. A comparison of six weeks with six months of oral anticoagulant therapy after a first episode of venous thromboembolism. Duration of Anticoagulation Trial Study Group. N Engl J Med 1995;332:1661–5.

31. Schulman S, Granqvist S, Holmström M, et al. The duration of oral anticoagulant therapy after a second episode of venous thromboembolism. The Duration of Anticoagulation Trial Study Group. N Engl J Med 1997;336:393–8.

32. Kearon C, Ginsberg JS, Kovacs MJ, et al.; Extended Low-Intensity Anticoagulation for Thrombo-Embolism Investigators. Comparison of low-intensity warfarin therapy with conventional-intensity warfarin therapy for long-term prevention of recurrent venous thromboembolism. N Engl J Med. 2003;349:631–9.

33. Ridker PM, Goldhaber SZ, Danielson E, et al.; PREVENT Investigators. Long-term, low-intensity warfarin therapy for the prevention of recurrent venous thromboembolism. N Engl J Med 2003;348:1425–34.

34. van Gogh Investigators, Buller HR, Cohen AT, et al. Idraparinux versus standard therapy for venous thromboembolic disease. N Engl J Med 2007;357:1094–104.

35. Elsharawy M, Elzayat E. Early results of thrombolysis vs anticoagulation in iliofemoral venous thrombosis. A randomised clinical trial. Eur J Vasc Endovasc Surg 2002;24:209–14.

36. Comerota AJ, Throm RC, Mathias SD, et al. Catheter-directed thrombolysis for iliofemoral deep venous thrombosis improves health-related quality of life. J Vasc Surg 2000;32:130–7.

37. Razavi MK, Wong H, Kee ST, et al. Initial clinical results of tenecteplase (TNK) in catheter-directed thrombolytic therapy. J Endovasc Ther 2002;9:593–8.

38. Plate G, Einarsson E, Ohlin P, et al. Thrombectomy with temporary arteriovenous fistula: the treatment of choice in acute iliofemoral venous thrombosis. J Vasc Surg 1984;1:867–76.

39. Decousus H, Leizorovicz A, Parent F, et al. A clinical trial of vena caval filters in the prevention of pulmonary embolism in patients with proximal deep-vein thrombosis. Prévention du Risque d'Embolie Pulmonaire par Interruption Cave Study Group. N Engl J Med 1998;338:409–15.

40. White RH, Zhou H, Kim J, Romano PS. A population-based study of the effectiveness of inferior vena cava filter use among patients with venous thromboembolism. Arch Intern Med 2000;160:2033–41.

41. Wan S, Quinlan DJ, Agnelli G, Eikelboom JW. Thrombolysis compared with heparin for the initial treatment of pulmonary embolism: a meta-analysis of the randomized controlled trials. Circulation 2004;110:744–9.

42. Büller HR, Agnelli G, Hull RD, et al. Antithrombotic therapy for venous thromboembolic disease: the Seventh ACCP Conference on Antithrombotic and Thrombolytic Therapy. Chest 2004;126:401–28S.

43. Kearon C, Kahn SR, Agnelli G, et al.; American College of Chest Physicians. Antithrombotic therapy for venous thromboembolic disease: American College of Chest Physicians Evidence-Based Clinical Practice Guidelines (8th Edition). Chest 2008;133:454–545S.

44. Otten HM, Prins MH. Venous thromboembolism and occult malignancy. Thromb Res 2001;102:V187–94.

45. Lloyd-Jones DM, Wang TJ, Leip EP, et al. Lifetime risk for development of atrial fibrillation: the Framingham heart study. Circulation 2004;110:1042–46.

46. Heeringa J, van der Kuip DA, Hofman A, et al. Prevalence, incidence and lifetime risk of atrial fibrillation: the Rotterdam study. Eur Heart J 2006;27:949–53.

47. Stewart S, Hart CL, Hole DJ, McMurray JJ. Population prevalence, incidence, and predictors of atrial fibrillation in the Renfrew/Paisley study. Heart 2001;86:516–21.

48. Miyasaka Y, Barnes ME, Gersh BJ, et al. Secular trends in incidence of atrial fibrillation in Olmsted County, Minnesota, 1980 to 2000, and implications on the projections for future prevalence. Circulation 2006;114:119–25.

49. Lip GY, Boss CJ. Antithrombotic treatment in atrial fibrillation. Heart 2006;92:155–61.

50. Fuster V, Rydén LE, Cannom DS, et al.; Cardiology/American Heart Association Task Force on Practice Guidelines and the European Society of Cardiology. ACC/AHA/ESC 2006 Guidelines for the management of patients with atrial fibrillation. J Am Coll Cardiol 2006;48:e149–246.

51. Klein AL, Jasper SE, Katz WE, et al.; ACUTE II Steering and Publications Committee for the ACUTE II Investigators. The use of enoxaparin compared with unfractionated heparin for short-term antithrombotic therapy in atrial fibrillation patients undergoing transoesophageal echocardiography-guided cardioversion: assessment of Cardioversion Using Transoesophageal Echocardiography (ACUTE) II randomized multicentre study. Eur Heart J 2006;27:2858–65.

52. Wu LA, Chandrasekaran K, Friedman PA, et al. Safety of expedited anticoagulation in patients undergoing transesophageal echocardiographic-guided cardioversion. Am J Med 2006;119:142–6.

53. Stroke Risk in Atrial Fibrillation Working Group. Independent predictors of stroke in patients with atrial fibrillation: a systematic review. Neurology 2007;69:546–54.

54. Hart RG, Pearce LA, Agullar MI. Antithrombotic therapy to prevent stroke in patients who have nonvalvular atrial fibrillation: a meta-analysis. Ann Intern Med 2007;146:857–67.

55. Lip GY, Edwards SJ. Stroke prevention with aspirin, warfarin and ximelagatran in patients with non-valvular atrial fibrillation: a systemic review and meta-analysis. Thromb Res 2006;118:321–33.

56. Stroke Prevention in Atrial Fibrillation investigators. A differential effect of aspirin in prevention of stroke on atrial fibrillation. J Stroke Cerebrovasc Dis 1993;3:181–8.

57. ACTIVE Writing Group on behalf of the ACTIVE Investigators. Clopidogrel plus aspirin versus oral anticoagulation for atrial fibrillation in the atrial fibrillation clopidogrel trial with irbesartan for prevention of vascular events (ACTIVE W). Lancet 2006;367:1903–12.

58. Mant J, Hobbs FD, Fletcher K, et al.; BAFTA investigators; Midland Research Practices Network (MidReC). Warfarin versus aspirin for stroke prevention in an elderly community population with atrial fibrillation (the Birmingham Atrial Fibrillation Treatment of the Aged Study, BAFTA): a randomised controlled trial. Lancet 2007;370:493–503.

59. Stein PD, Alpert JS, Bussey HI, et al. Antithrombotic therapy in patients with mechanical and biological prosthetic heart valves. Chest. 2001;119:220–7S.

60. American College of Cardiology/American Heart Association Task Force on Practice Guidelines; Society of Cardiovascular Anesthesiologists; Society for Cardiovascular Angiography and Interventions; Society of Thoracic Surgeons, Bonow RO, Carabello BA, Kanu C, et al. ACC/AHA 2006 guidelines for the management of patients with valvular heart disease: a report of the American College of Cardiology/American Heart Association Task Force on Practice Guidelines (writing committee to revise the 1998 Guidelines for the Management of Patients With Valvular Heart Disease): developed in collaboration with the Society of Cardiovascular Anesthesiologists: endorsed by the Society for Cardiovascular Angiography and Interventions and the Society of Thoracic Surgeons. Circulation 2006;114:e84–231.

61. Vaitkus PT. Left ventricular mural thrombus and the risk of embolic stroke after acute myocardial infarction. J Cardiovasc Risk 1995;2:103–6.

62. Loh E, Sutton MS, Wun CC, et al. Ventricular dysfunction and the risk of stroke after myocardial infarction. N Engl J Med 1997;336:251–7.

63. Antman EM, Anbe DT, Armstrong PW, et al. ACC/AHA Guidelines for the Management of Patients With ST-Elevation Myocardial Infarction – Executive summary: a report of the American College of Cardiology/American Heart Association Task Force on Practice Guidelines (Writing Committee to Revise the 1999 Guidelines for the Management of Patients with Acute Myocardial Infarction). Circulation 2004;110:588–636.

64. Tangelder MJ, Frison L, Weaver D, et al. Effect of ximelagatran on ischemic events and death in patients with atrial fibrillation after acute myocardial infarction in the efficacy and safety of the oral direct thrombin inhibitor ximelagatran in patients with recent myocardial damage (ESTEEM) trial. Am Heart J 2008;155:382–7.

65. Coumadin Aspirin Refarction Study (CARS) Investigators. Randomised double-blind trial of fixed low dose warfarin with aspirin after myocardial infarction. Lancet 1997;350:389–96.

66. Fiore L, Ezekowitz MD, Brophy MT, et al. Department of Veterans Affairs Cooperative Studies Program Clinical Trial comparing combined warfarin and aspirin with aspirin alone in survivors of acute myocardial infarction: primary results of the CHAMP study. Circulation 2002;105:557–63.

67. Hurlen M, Abdelnoor M, Smith P, et al. Warfarin, aspirin or both after myocardial infarction. N Engl J Med 2002;347:969–74.

68. Van Es RF, Jonker JJC, Verheugt FWA, et al. Aspirin and coumadin after acute coronary syndromes (the ASPECT-2 study). Lancet 2002;360:109–13.

69. Lip GYH, Karpha M. Anticoagulant and antiplatelet therapy use in patients with atrial fibrillation undergoing percutaneous coronary intervention: the need for consensus and a management guideline. Chest 2006;130:1823–7.

70. Lip GY, Gibbs CR. Antiplatelet agents versus control or anticoagulation for heart failure in sinus rhythm: a Cochrane systematic review. Q J Med 2002;95:461–8.
71. Lip GYH, Gibbs CR. Anticoagulation for heart failure in sinus rhythm: a Cochrane systemic review. Q J Med 2002;95:451–9.
72. Cleland JG, Findlay I, Jafri S, et al. The Warfarin/Aspirin Study in Heart Failure (WASH): a randomised trial comparing antithrombotic strategies for patients with heart failure. Am Heart J 2004;148:157–64.
73. Massie BM, Krol WF, Ammon SE, et al. The Warfarin and Antiplatelet Therapy in Heart Failure trial (WATCH): rationale, design, and baseline patient characteristics. J Card Fail 2004;10:101–12.
74. Warfarin versus Aspirin in Reduced Cardiac Ejection Fraction (WARCEF). www.clinicaltrials.gov, Identifier: NCT00041938
75. Petersen P, Boysen G, Godtfredsen J, et al. Placebo-controlled, randomised trial of warfarin and aspirin for prevention of thromboembolic complications in chronic atrial fibrillation. The Copenhagen AFASAK study. Lancet 1989;i:175–9.
76. The Boston Area Anticoagulation Trial for Atrial Fibrillation Investigators. The effect of low-dose warfarin on the risk of stroke in patients with nonrheumatic atrial fibrillation. N Engl J Med 1990;323:1505–11.
77. Connolly SJ, Laupacis A, Gent M, et al. Canadian Atrial Fibrillation Anticoagulation (CAFA) Study. J Am Coll Cardiol 1991;18:349–55.
78. Secondary prevention in non-rheumatic atrial fibrillation after transient ischaemic attack or minor stroke. EAFT (European Atrial Fibrillation Trial) Study Group. Lancet 1993;342:1255–62.
79. Stroke Prevention in Atrial Fibrillation Study. Final results. Circulation 1991;84:527–39.
80. Ezekowitz MD, Bridgers SL, James KE, et al. Warfarin in the prevention of stroke associated with nonrheumatic atrial fibrillation. Veterans Affairs Stroke Prevention in Nonrheumatic Atrial Fibrillation Investigators. N Engl J Med 1992;327:1406–12.
81. Diener HC, Cunha L, Forbes C, et al. European Stroke Prevention Study. 2. Dipyridamole and acetylsalicylic acid in the secondary prevention of stroke. J Neurol Sci 1996;143:1–13.
82. Benavente O, Hart R, Koudstaal P, et al. Antiplatelet therapy for preventing stroke in patients with non-valvular atrial fibrillation and no previous history of stroke or transient ischemic attacks. Cochrane Database Syst Rev 2000;(2):CD001925.
83. Japan Atrial Fibrillation Stroke Trial Group. Low-dose aspirin for prevention of stroke in low-risk patients with atrial fibrillation: Japan Atrial Fibrillation Stoke Trial. Stroke 2006;37:447–51.
84. Posada IS, Barriales V. Alternate-day dosing of aspirin in atrial fibrillation. LASAF Pilot Study Group. Am Heart J 1999;138:137–43.

Chapter 3

The vitamin K antagonists and their limitations

Chee W Khoo, Gregory YH Lip

The vitamin K antagonists (VKAs) have been the mainstay of oral anticoagulant therapy for more than 50 years, warfarin being the VKA most commonly used worldwide. The longstanding popularity of the VKAs is largely based on their effectiveness in the prevention and treatment of venous thromboembolism (VTE), as well as the prevention of systemic embolism in patients who have mechanical heart valves or atrial fibrillation (AF).

Pharmacology of warfarin

The pharmacological effects of warfarin are based on its ability to inhibit the activity of vitamin K-dependent coagulation factors (factors II, VII, IX and X). To express their procoagulant activity these factors require γ-carboxylation, a process dependent on the availability of vitamin K, which in turn depends on normal functioning of the enzyme vitamin K epoxide reductase. Inhibition of this enzyme by warfarin causes a lack of vitamin K and consequently results in the production of functionally impaired, partially carboxylated and decarboxylated factors, with corresponding anticoagulant effects [1].

As well as their anticoagulant effect, VKAs also have procoagulant potential via prevention of carboxylation of anticoagulant proteins C and S. However, as a rule, the anticoagulation effects of VKAs outweigh their pro-coagulant properties.

Warfarin consists of a racemic mixture of two optically active isomers, the *R* and *S* forms. The *S*-isomer is five times more potent than the *R*-isomer with respect to vitamin K antagonism [2].

There is substantial variability in the oral absorption and bioavailability of warfarin due to its multiple interactions with dietary constituents, lifestyle factors and concomitant drugs. For example, the administration of low-dose vitamin K can reverse the effect of warfarin, whereas high concentrations of vitamin K may result in its accumulation in the liver and make the patient resistant to warfarin for a prolonged period of time. Genetic factors also play a role in a patient's response to warfarin (see below). Because of the interplay of all these characteristics, substantial inter- and intra-individual variability in dosing is typical of VKAs.

Warfarin is mainly bound to albumin in the plasma and metabolised by the liver. It has a relatively long half-life of around 40 hours. This means it often takes several days to reach therapeutic level of the drug. Figure 3.1 summarises its main pharmacological characteristics.

Pharmacological characteristics of warfarin	
Target on coagulation cascade	Vitamin K episode reductase
Prodrug	No
Dosing	Variable
Bioavailability	Variable
Time to peak drug level	Variable
Half-life (h)	40
Route of elimination	Metabolisation in liver
Renal clearance (%)	0
Interaction	Polypharmacy, dietary vitamin K
Safety in pregnancy	No
Antidote	Vitamin K

Figure 3.1 Pharmacological characteristics of warfarin.

Pharmacogenetics of warfarin

Polymorphisms of two genes, *CYP450 2C9* and *VKORC1*, have been identified as playing major roles in warfarin activity. CYP450 2C9 is involved in the oxidative metabolism of the potent S-isomer of warfarin [3], and mutations are independently associated with an abnormal response to warfarin. *CYP450 2C9* polymorphism explains about 10% of the variation in warfarin dosing among white Europeans, and it is relatively rare in Asian and African American populations [4].

About 25% of the dosing variation between individuals is attributable to *VKORC1* polymorphism. Two main haplotypes have been identified in a north American study: low-dose haplotype group A and high-dose haplotype group B [5]. In patients with the group A haplotype, which was mainly found in Asian-Americans, there was more rapid achievement of the therapeutic range. In contrast, patients with group B haplotype, which was mainly found in African-Americans, were relatively resistant to warfarin.

Interactions of warfarin with other drugs and food

Various commonly used medications, diets and comorbidities have been shown to interact with warfarin, accounting for much of the inter- and intra-individual variability in therapeutic dosing.

The drugs known to interact with warfarin are mainly inducers and inhibitors of CYP450 2C9 [6], an enzyme responsible for the metabolism of the potent S-isomer of warfarin. CYP450 2C9 inhibitors include amiodarone, fluconazole, isoniazid and sertraline. Rifampicin and barbiturates are known to induce CYP450 2C9. Other enzymes, such as CYP1A2 and CYP3A4, are responsible for the metabolism of the R-isomer. The quinolones, macrolides, metronidazole and fluconazole inhibit these enzymes. Commonly used drugs that inhibit liver enzymes and potentiate the effect of warfarin are summarised in Figure 3.2. Commonly used drugs that induce liver enzymes and inhibit the effect of warfarin are summarised in Figure 3.3.

Interactions of other drugs with warfarin relate to serum protein binding. Warfarin is highly protein bound in the serum. Other highly protein-bound drugs can displace warfarin from serum albumin and potentiate its anticoagulant effect [7].

Drugs with enzyme-inhibiting properties that enhance warfarin effects		
Anti-infective	**Cardiovascular**	**Others**
Ciprofloxacin	Amiodarone	Citalopram
Erythromycin	Diltiazem	Sertraline
Co-trimoxazole	Fenofibrate	Entacapone
Fluconazole	Propafenone	Alcohol
Isoniazid	Propranolol	Disulfiram
Metronidazole	Quinidine	Phenytoin
Miconazole		Cimetidine

Figure 3.2 Drugs with enzyme-inhibiting properties that enhance warfarin's effects.

Drugs with enzyme-inducing properties that inhibit warfarin effects		
Anti-infective	**Central nervous system**	**Others**
Rifampicin	Barbiturates	Mercaptopurine
Ribavirin	Carbamazepine	Mesalazine
	Chlordiazepoxide	Azathioprine

Figure 3.3 Drugs with enzyme-inducing properties that inhibit warfarin's effects.

Foods that contain a high level of vitamin K, for example broccoli, reduce the effect of warfarin. Excessive use of alcohol, which interferes with liver enzymes, may also affect the metabolism of warfarin [6]. Additionally, some herbs have been found to modify the effects of warfarin; for example St John's wort (used for treatment of depression) may reduce the anticoagulant effect [6].

Commencement of anticoagulation

Following administration of warfarin, newly synthesised, dysfunctional, vitamin K-dependent clotting factors gradually replace the normal clotting factors. However, the rate of replacement of each of the different factors varies substantially, and the full anticoagulant effect of warfarin is often delayed. Importantly, as well as being time-dependent, this effect also depends on the dose administered. Of note, it has occasionally been reported that prompt loading with high doses of warfarin may trigger blockade of the anticoagulant proteins C and S before the inhibition of coagulation factors commences, thus causing a brief and transitional rise in prothrombotic risk. However, the clinical relevance of this phenomenon has not been established an for patients who do not require rapid anticoagulation, a slow-loading regimen may be safer.

The majority of patients achieve therapeutic anticoagulation within 3–4 days [8,9]. If rapid anticoagulation is needed, a higher loading dose of warfarin or concomitant heparin injections can be used, accompanied by daily monitoring of the international normalised ratio (INR).

Monitoring of warfarin therapy
Prothrombin time and INR

The large number of pharmacological interactions of warfarin and the risk of severe haemorrhagic complications mandate thorough monitoring of its anticoagulant activity. Prothrombin time (PT) used to be the most common test used to monitor VKAs. However, PT reporting could not be standardised because it was measured using reagents that had variable sensitivity. The results were expressed in seconds or as a simple ratio of patient:normal PT. The results were often not comparable between different laboratories, and this led to confusion regarding the appropriate therapeutic range and dose of warfarin.

A better calibrated model, the INR, was adopted in 1982 [10]. The INR is the ratio of measured PT over mean normal PT, using a specific reagent of known sensitivity. INR is more reliable than the unconverted PT ratio [11]. Hence, it is recommended for use in the initiation and monitoring of warfarin therapy. The recommended targets of INR for oral anticoagulant therapy have been well studied and are summarised in Figure 3.4 [8].

In clinical practice, a therapeutic range is often used rather than a single target because the INR is highly variable. Thus, a target INR of 2.5 implies a therapeutic range of 2.0–3.0, whereas a target INR of 3.0 signifies a therapeutic range of 2.5–3.5.

Indications for oral anticoagulation and target international normalised ratio	
Indication	**Target INR**
Pulmonary embolism (PE)	2.5
Deep vein thrombosis (DVT)	2.5
Recurrence PE/DVT when not on warfarin	2.5
Recurrence PE/DVT when on warfarin	3.5
Non-valvular atrial fibrillation	2.5
Electrical cardioversion	2.5
Symptomatic inherited thrombophilia	2.5
Mural thrombus	2.5
Cardiomyopathy	2.5
Aortic mechanical heart valve	2.5–3.5*
Mitral mechanical heart valve	3.0 – 3.5*

Figure 3.4 Indications for oral anticoagulation and target international normalised ratio.
* Depending on types of valve implanted.

The effectiveness and safety of warfarin are critically dependent on maintaining the INR within the therapeutic range. In order to achieve this, a monitoring system has to be in place.

Approaches to INR monitoring

The traditional model of care for patients who take oral anticoagulants requires regular attendance at an anticoagulation clinic for INR monitoring. This service usually requires input from a physician, pathologist, specialist nurse or even a pharmacist. A venous blood sample or capillary blood sample is used. If the INR result cannot be reported immediately, the patient receives dosing and recall advice through the post or by telephone. If the INR result is available when the patient is present, a dosing recommendation can be made and the patient can be given a date for his or her next appointment. This cycle is continued for as long as the patient needs anticoagulation.

Some general practices have set up anticoagulation services in the community. They either obtain a venous sample and then make dosing recommendations and give recall advice once the INR result becomes available, or they use 'near-patient' or 'point-of-care' testing, with or without computer-assisted dosing.

An increasing number of patients are using near-patient or point-of-care coagulation monitoring devices for self-monitoring of long-term oral anticoagulant therapy. A systemic review of 14 randomised controlled trials of self-monitoring has shown that self-monitoring alone significantly reduced thromboembolic events, major haemorrhage and all-cause mortality [12]. Self-monitoring of INR provides an alternative to clinic-based monitoring. However, it requires appropriate infrastructure within the healthcare system to support the service.

INR monitoring is a difficult task, partly due to the high variability and narrow therapeutic window. One study conducted in a university teaching hospital and involving 2,223 patients with atrial fibrillation showed that almost a third of the treatment time and close to half of the INR readings were outside the therapeutic range [13].

It is not surprising that INR monitoring comprises a significant burden for healthcare systems. This might explain why oral anticoagulation therapy is still suboptimal despite well-publicised guidelines. There is physician reluctance to prescribe oral anticoagulation therapy, as reflected by the Euro Heart Survey finding that only 67% of patients eligible for the therapy were actually prescribed it [14]. This is dicussed in more detail in Chapter 4.

Conclusions

Until recently, VKAs were the only choice for oral anticoagulation, warfarin being the most commonly used VKA worldwide. However, the utility of warfarin is limited by its narrow therapeutic window and slow onset and offset of action, as well as by substantial inter- and intra-individual variability in the therapeutic dose, which all necessitate regular dose adjustment to keep within the therapeutic range. Furthermore, the metabolism of warfarin is also influenced by genetic polymorphisms and by dietary and numerous drug interactions. All these factors have made INR monitoring a difficult task.

References

1. Malhotra OP, Nesheim ME, Mann KG. The kinetics of activation of normal and gamma carboxy glutamic acid deficient prothrombins. J Biol Chem 1985;260:279–87.
2. Hirsh J, Fuster V, Ansell J, Halperin JL; American Heart Association/American College of Cardiology Foundation. American Heart Association/American College of Cardiology Foundation guide to warfarin therapy. J Am Coll Cardiol 2003;41:1633–52.
3. Mannucci PM. Genetic control of anticoagulation. Lancet 1999;353:688–9.
4. Sanderson S, Emery J, Higgins J. CYP2C9 gene variants, drug dose, and bleeding risk in warfarin-treated patients: a HuGEnet systematic review and meta-analysis. Genet Med 2005;7:97–104.
5. Rieder MJ, Reiner AP, Gage BF, et al. Effect of VKORC1 haplotypes on transcriptional regulation and warfarin dose. N Engl J Med 2005;352:2285–93.
6. Holbrook AM, Pereira JA, Labiris R, et al. Systematic overview of warfarin and its drug and food interaction. Arch Intern Med 2005;165:1095–106.
7. Gage BF, Fihn SD, White RH. Management and dosing of warfarin therapy. Am J Med 2000;109:481–8.
8. Baglin TP, Keeling DM, Watson HG. Guidelines on oral anticoagulation (warfarin): third edition – 2005 update. Br J Haematol 2006;132:277–85.
9. Hirsh J, Dalen J, Anderson DR, et al. Oral anticoagulants: mechanism of action, clinical effectiveness, and optimal therapeutic range. Chest 2001;119(suppl):8–21S.
10. Kirkwood TBL. Calibration of reference thromboplastins and standardisation of the prothrombin time ratio. Thromb Haemost 1983;49:238–44.
11. Johnston M, Harrison L, Moffat K, et al. Reliability of the international normalized ratio for monitoring the induction phase of warfarin: comparison with the prothrombin time ratio. J Lab Clin Med 1996;128:214–17.
12. Heneghan C, Alonso-Coello P, Garcia-Alamino JM, et al. Self-monitoring of oral anticoagulation: a systemic review and meta-analysis. Lancet 2006;367:404–11.
13. Jones M, McEwan P, Morgan CL, et al. Evaluation of the pattern of treatment, level of anticoagulation control, and outcome of treatment with warfarin in patients with non-valvular atrial fibrillation: a record linkage study in a large British population. Heart 2005; 91:472–7.
14. Nieuwlaat R, Capucci A, Lip GY, et al.; Euro Heart Survey Investigators. Antithrombotic treatment in real-life atrial fibrillation patients: a report from the Euro Heart Survey on Atrial Fibrillation. Eur Heart J 2006;27:3018–26.

References

Chapter 4

Haemorrhage risks, patient perspectives, and quality-of-life issues

Kok-Hoon Tay, Deirdre A Lane, Gregory YH Lip

It is estimated that, in the UK, for example, 950,000 patients are currently taking warfarin (2% of the general practice population). This number is expected to rise by approximately 10% per annum, primarily because of its use in AF [1].

Commencing warfarin is not without its risks and complications. Warfarin has diverse pharmacokinetics and pharmacodynamics in different patients, which result in the need for individual dose-adjustment based on the international normalised ratio (INR). Monitoring to maintain anticoagulation within the therapeutic range is essential to minimise the results of warfarin-related complications, such as haemorrhage or thromboembolic events. Furthermore, it is also required because the INR is affected by a number of medications (antibiotics, especially macrolides/quinolones, antifungals, anticonvulsants such as phenytoin, non-steroidal anti-inflammatory drugs, amiodarone) and by alcohol, herbal medicines and foods high in vitamin K, as already discussed in Chapter 3.

There are a multitude of physician- and patient-related factors that lead to under-utilisation of oral anticoagulant therapy. Along with the risk of haemorrhage, these are discussed below.

Risk of haemorrhage

The most common side-effect from warfarin is haemorrhage from any anatomical site. The most feared complication from over-anticoagulation (INR >3.0) is intracranial haemorrhage, which accounts for approximately 90% of deaths from warfarin-associated haemorrhage and for the majority of disability among survivors [2]. Moreover, the benefit of warfarin is only conferred upon atrial fibrillation (AF) patients if the minimum percentage of time spent within the therapeutic INR range is between 58 and 65% [3]. Given the inherent difficulties associated with warfarin control, initiating warfarin is not always a straightforward decision, especially in elderly patients in whom the situation is usually compounded by multiple comorbidities, which further increase the risk of haemorrhage.

Nonetheless, intracranial haemorrhage rates in clinical trials conducted in AF patients on oral anticoagulant therapy are small, reported to be between 0.3 and 0.6% per year [4], and the absolute increase in major extracranial haemorrhages is even smaller, at ≤0.3% per year [5]. It may be that these figures reflect better-quality INR monitoring and greater intensity of intervention by anticoagulation services in clinical trials, and outside the research setting the actual figures may be higher.

However, with careful INR monitoring and dose adjustment of oral anticoagulant therapy, warfarin can significantly reduce the risk of cardioembolic stroke: 64% (95% confidence interval [CI] 49–74%) compared to placebo, and 39% (95% CI 22–52%) compared with antiplatelet agents [6]. The risk of intracranial haemorrhage associated with warfarin use was twice that of aspirin but the absolute risk was small at 0.2% per year [6]. Furthermore, among elderly patients (>75 years), the rate of major haemorrhage in aspirin users (2.0% per year) does not differ significantly from warfarin users (1.9% per year), as evidenced by the Birmingham Atrial Fibrillation of the Aged (BAFTA) study [7].

Risk factors for haemorrhage

There are many risk factors that increase the risk of haemorrhage in patients on oral anticoagulant therapy, such as:

- increasing age (≥60),
- previous stroke
- comorbidities, i.e. diabetes mellitus, recent myocardial infarction, anaemia (defined as haematocrit <30%), presence of malignancy, concomitant antiplatelet usage, uncontrolled hypertension, liver/renal failure and previous gastrointestinal bleed.

Many of the risk factors for haemorrhage are also risk factors for stroke, and therefore the decision as to whether to commence oral anticoagulation should be highly individualised [8]. There are numerous stroke risk stratification schema to assist decision-making in prescribing oral anticoagulant therapy for AF patients, such as the $CHADS_2$ [Congestive heart failure, Hypertension, Age >75, Diabetes mellitus and previous stroke] schema, and other schemata from the American College of Cardiology (ACC), American College of Chest Physicians (ACCP), American Heart Association (AHA), European Society of

Cardiology (ESC) and UK National Institute for Health and Clinical Excellence (NICE). In contrast, however, there is currently no universal haemorrhage risk stratification schema commonly employed in clinical practice.

To date, four haemorrhage risk predictor schemata have been proposed (Figure 4.1) [9–12]. All four utilise age as one of the consistent predictors of haemorrhage risks, albeit with varying age categories: Kuijer et al. [10] use age ≥60 (lowest age) whereas Gage et al. [12] use age >75 (highest age). Only the Kuijer et al. [10] and Shireman et al. [11] models include female sex as a risk factor for haemorrhage when on warfarin. Previous significant haemorrhage and anaemia (defined as haematocrit <30%) are regarded as important risk factors in all models [9,11,12] except that of Kuijer et al. [10]. Other comorbid risk factors taken into account in the four schemata include previous history of stroke, liver/renal failure, presence of diabetes mellitus, antiplatelet usage, uncontrolled hypertension, thrombocytopenia, excessive falls, alcohol abuse, recent myocardial infarction and haemorrhagic events (within 3 months).

Collectively, these four haemorrhage risk models were derived from studies of patients who were on warfarin for numerous reasons and not just for AF, for instance including patients who had valvular heart surgery, deep vein thrombosis (DVT), pulmonary embolism (PE), stroke, transient ischaemic attack or other thromboembolism. Only the two most recent schemata [11,12] were drawn from populations consisting exclusively of AF patients. It is worth noting that these four haemorrhage risk predictor models were mainly derived from white patients, and the risk factors may not necessarily translate to non-white patients. Hence, there is very little consensus on the risk factors included within these schemata, and they lack clinical validation in an AF population. Consequently their predictive value is unknown, limiting their widespread clinical application [13].

Physician barriers to use of warfarin

Despite the wealth of evidence for the superiority of warfarin over aspirin in thromboprophylaxis to minimise stroke risk in AF (relative risk reduction [RRR] 39%, 95% CI 22–52%) [6], the Euro Heart Survey demonstrated that only 67% of eligible AF patients are actually prescribed oral anticoagulant therapy [14]. Physicians' reluctance to prescribe warfarin is often due to a misperception of the magnitude of the risk of haemorrhage, overestimation of the associated risks, underestimation of the stroke risk and clinical uncertainty or inexperience with warfarin [15]. Physicians who have more experience with warfarin or longer-standing practices tend to be more willing to prescribe it than their younger, less experienced counterparts [16,17].

Published haemorrhage risk schemata				
Study	Low	Moderate	High	Risk factors for score calculation
Beyth et al. [9]	0	1–2	≥ 3	Age ≥ 65 years, gastrointestinal bleed in 2 weeks, previous stroke, comorbidities (1 of 4 – recent myocardial infarction, anaemia, diabetes mellitus and renal impairment), with 1 point for presence of each condition and 0 for absence.
Kuijer et al. [10]	0	1–3	> 3	Risk score = [1.6 x age] + [1.3 x sex] + [2.2 x malignancy], with 1 point for being ≥60, female or presence of malignancy and 0 for absence
Shireman et al. [11]	≤ 1.07	>1.07 but <2.19	≥ 2.19	Risk score = [0.49 x age] + [0.32 x female] + [0.58 x remote bleed] + [0.62 x recent bleed] + [0.71 x alcohol/drug abuse] + [0.27 x diabetes] + [0.86 x anaemia] + [0.32 x antiplatelet], with 1 point for presence of each condition and 0 for absence
Gage et al. [12]	0–1	2–3	≥ 4	Hepatic/renal disease, alcohol abuse, malignancy, older (age > 75 years), ↓ platelet count, rebleeding risk, uncontrolled hypertension, anaemia, genetic factor, excessive falls, stroke, with 2 points given to previous bleed and 1 point to each of the other factors

Figure 4.1. Published haemorrhage risk schemata. Adapted with permission from Tay et al. [13].

A national survey conducted among Australian family physicians treating non-valvular AF patients revealed that a higher percentage of the GPs reported a stroke in a patient who was not on an oral anticoagulant than reported an intracranial haemorrhage in a patient who was on an oral anticoagulant (45.8% vs 15.8%) [17]. Despite this, a physician's exposure to adverse events such as haemorrhage may play an exaggerated role in treatment decisions. Indeed, one study reported that adverse outcomes from anticoagulation have a greater influence on management decisions than occurrences of avoidable ischaemic stroke: the odds of a physician prescribing warfarin were reduced after exposure to a patient who had serious haemorrhage when taking warfarin, but they were not changed after exposure to a patient who had thromboembolic event while not taking warfarin [18].

Patient barriers to use of warfarin

In contrast, patients are more concerned with reducing the risk of ischaemic stroke [19]. Hence they are more accepting of warfarin and its inherent problems (life-long monitoring of INR, and interactions with food, alcohol and drugs), and of the associated risk of haemorrhage, in order to avoid an ischaemic stroke and its consequences [16].

Nevertheless, there are patient barriers to warfarin prescription, the most pertinent of which are patients' often limited knowledge about the disease, its treatment and the risk–benefit ratio of warfarin thromboprophylaxis [20], and their preferences for treatment [15]. It is important to involve patients in the decision-making process of whether or not to initiate warfarin [21]. Research has demonstrated that patients who are well-informed about treatment regimens are less anxious and more satisfied with treatment, and have higher rates of compliance and better outcomes [22]. Patient preferences for treatment need to be considered, given that the success of thromboprophylactic therapy and avoidance of warfarin-related complications rely largely on the patients' adherence to the warfarin regimen, complying with regular INR monitoring and taking into account drug, food and alcohol interactions. A study of patients' preferences for anticoagulant treatment revealed that two out of five patients would prefer not to receive it, which may be due to misconceptions about anticoagulants and patients' lack of understanding of the reduction in stroke risk associated with anticoagulation [21]. A brief educational intervention demonstrated an improvement in patients' knowledge of AF and the need for anticoagulation, and the factors affecting INR control [23].

Quality of life in atrial fibrillation

As discussed in Chapter 2, warfarin remains the most efficacious prophylaxis for AF patients who have at least moderate risk of stroke. The development of AF in any patient and its subsequent treatment can encroach on aspects of patients' quality of life (QoL). AF may give the impression of being a benign cardiac arrhythmia but it can be a disabling heart disease with complications related to the treatment strategy, be it 'rate control' or 'rhythm control', which impact negatively on quality of life.

There have been many studies conducted assessing the impact of interventional/non-interventional treatment strategies for rate/rhythm control on QoL in AF patients [24]. QoL is impaired in patients with AF compared with healthy controls [25]. It has been demonstrated that QoL can be significantly improved by either rate or rhythm control, but there does not appear to be a clear benefit of one treatment modality over the other in terms of QoL. Two randomised controlled trials (AFFIRM [26] and RACE [25]) compared QoL directly for rate and rhythm strategies, rather than changes within each strategy from baseline. Both studies found no significant differences between rhythm and rate control in any of the QoL subscales on the Short Form-36 health survey questionnaires. However, most AF patients report a significant improvement in QoL after having had atrioventricular (AV) node ablation with or without pacing, radiofrequency catheter ablation/pulmonary vein isolation and the Maze operation [24], and this is probably due to the reduction in, or resolution of, symptoms following these interventions.

Another important consideration is the impact of oral anticoagulant therapy on QoL in AF patients. It appears that treatment strategy – 'rate or rhythm control' – exerts more influence over QoL than anticoagulation therapy. A cross-sectional study conducted in 330 elderly (>75 years) AF patients revealed that long-term warfarin (>1 year) itself did not affect their physical or mental QoL compared with the general elderly population [27]. Likewise, there is no change in QoL in a younger AF population (mean age 68 years) either, as demonstrated in the North American study, Boston Area Anticoagulation Trial for Atrial Fibrillation (BAATAF) [28].

Conclusions

All in all, when physicians are faced with a newly diagnosed AF patient, a wide spectrum of factors needs to be considered, in addition to management of the AF itself. Patients' perceptions about the disease and its treatment need to be assessed. Patients need to be encouraged to be active participants in their own healthcare. The success of treatment – of rate or rhythm control and of anticoagulation – requires patient adherence to a revised lifestyle regimen.

Currently, the complexities involved in managing warfarin treatment (regular INR checks, and awareness of drug, food and alcohol interactions) mean that not all eligible patients are prescribed it, due to safety and compliance concerns. With the advent of novel anticoagulants, such as direct oral thrombin inhibitors (ie, dabigatran) or factor Xa inhibitors (apixaban, rivaroxaban, DU176b, YM150), some of the inherent problems, such as regular INR monitoring and dose adjustment, and drug, food, and alcohol interactions, will be removed, hopefully enabling more eligible patients to receive oral anticoagulant therapy.

References

1. Connock M, Stevens C, Fry-Smith A, et al. Clinical effectiveness and cost-effectiveness of different models of managing long-term oral anticoagulation therapy: a systematic review and economic modeling. Health Technol Assess 2007;11:iii–iv, ix–66.

2. Fang MC, Go AS, Chang Y, et al. Death and disability from warfarin-associated intracranial and extracranial haemorrhages. Am J Med 2007;120:700–5.

3. Connolly SJ, Pogue J, Eikelboom J, et al.; ACTIVE W Investigators. Benefit of oral anticoagulant over antiplatelet therapy in atrial fibrillation depends on the quality of international normalized ratio control achieved by centers and countries as measured by time in therapeutic range. Circulation 2008;118:2029–37.

4. Hart RG, Tonarelli SB, Pearce LA. Avoiding central nervous system bleeding during antithrombotic therapy: recent data and ideas. Stroke 2005;36:1588–93.

5. Lip GY, Lim HS. Atrial fibrillation and stroke prevention. Lancet Neurol 2007;6:981–993.

6. Hart RG, Pearce LA, Aguilar MI. Meta-analysis: antithrombotic therapy to prevent stroke in patients who have nonvalvular atrial fibrillation. Ann Intern Med 2007;146:857–67

7. Mant J, Hobbs FD, Fletcher K, et al.; BAFTA investigators; Midland Research Practices Network (MidReC). Warfarin versus aspirin for stroke prevention in an elderly community population with atrial fibrillation (the Birmingham Atrial Fibrillation Treatment of the Aged Study, BAFTA): a randomised controlled trial. Lancet 2007;370:493–503.

8. Poli D, Antonucci E, Marcucci R, et al. Risk of bleeding in very old atrial fibrillation patients on warfarin: relationship with ageing and CHADS$_2$ score. Thromb Res 2007;121:347–52.

9. Beyth RJ, Quinn LM, Landefeld CS. Prospective evaluation of an index for predicting the risk of major bleeding in outpatients treated with warfarin. Am J Med 1998;105:91–9.

10. Kuijer PMM, Hutten BA, Prins MH, Büller HR. Prediction of the risk of bleeding during anticoagulant treatment for venous thromboembolism. Arch Intern Med 1999;159:457–60.

11. Shireman TI, Mahnken JD, Howard PA, et al. Development of a contemporary bleeding risk model for elderly warfarin recipients. Chest 2006;130:1390–6.

12. Gage BF, Yan Y, Milligan PE, et al. Clinical classification schemes for predicting haemorrhage: Results from the National Registry of Atrial Fibrillation (NRAF). Am Heart J 2006;151:713–19.

13. Tay KH, Lane DA, Lip GY. Bleeding risks with combination of oral anticoagulation plus antiplatelet therapy: is clopidogrel any safer than aspirin when combined with warfarin? Thromb Haemost 2008;100:955–7.

14. Nieuwlaat R, Capucci A, Lip GY, et al.; Euro Heart Survey Investigators. Antithrombotic treatment in real-life atrial fibrillation patients: a report from the Euro Heart Survey on Atrial Fibrillation. Eur Heart J 2006;27:3018–26.

15. Lane DA, Lip GY. Barriers to anticoagulation in patients with atrial fibrillation: changing physician-related factors. Stroke 2008;39:7–9.

16. Bungard TJ, Ghali WA, Teo KK, et al. Why do patients with atrial fibrillation not receive warfarin? Arch Intern Med 2000;160:41–6.

17. Gattellari M, Worthington J, Zwar N, Middleton S. Barriers to the use of anticoagulation for nonvalvular atrial fibrillation: a representative survey of Australian family physicians. Stroke 2008;39:227–30.

18. Choudhry NK, Anderson GM, Laupacis A, et al. Impact of adverse events on prescribing warfarin in patients with atrial fibrillation: matched pair analysis. BMJ 2006;332:141–5.

19. Devereaux PJ, Anderson DR, Gardner MJ, et al. Differences between perspectives of physicians and patients on anticoagulation in patients with atrial fibrillation: observational study. BMJ 2001;323:1218–22.

20. Lip GY, Agnelli G, Thach AA, et al. Oral anticoagulation in atrial fibrillation: A pan-European patient survey. Eur J Intern Med 2007;18:202–8.

21. Protheroe J, Fahey T, Montgomery AA, Peters TJ. The impact of patients' preferences on the treatment of atrial fibrillation: observational study of patient based decision analysis. BMJ 2000;320:1380–4.

22. Lane D, Lip GY. Anti-thrombotic therapy for atrial fibrillation and patients' preferences for treatment. Age Ageing 2005;34:1–3.

23. Lane DA, Ponsford J, Shelley A, et al. Patient knowledge and perceptions of atrial fibrillation and anticoagulant therapy: effects of an educational intervention programme. The West Birmingham Atrial Fibrillation Project. Int J Cardiol 2006;110:354–58.

24. Thrall G, Lane D, Carroll D, Lip GY. Quality of life in patients with atrial fibrillation: a systematic review. Am J Med 2006;119:448.e1–19.

25. Hagens VE, Ranchor AV, Van Sonderen E, et al.; RACE Study Group. Effect of rate or rhythm control on quality of life in persistent atrial fibrillation. Results from the Rate Control Versus Electrical Cardioversion (RACE) Study. J Am Coll Cardiol 2004;43:241–7.

26. Jenkins LS, Brodsky M, Schron E, et al. Quality of life in atrial fibrillation: the Atrial Fibrillation Follow-up Investigation of Rhythm Management (AFFIRM) study. Am Heart J 2005;149:112–20.

27. Das AK, Willcoxson PD, Corrado OJ, West RM. The impact of long-term warfarin on the quality of life of elderly people with atrial fibrillation. Age Ageing 2007;36:95–7.

28. Lancaster TR, Singer DE, Sheehan MA, et al. The impact of long-term warfarin therapy on quality of life. Evidence from a randomized trial. Boston Area Anticoagulation Trial for Atrial Fibrillation Investigators. Arch Intern Med 1991;151:1944–9.

Chapter 5

New oral anticoagulants

Direct thrombin inhibitors

Eduard Shantsila, Gregory YH Lip

Anticoagulation can be achieved by inhibition of the various coagulation factors. For example, as discussed in the preceding chapters, warfarin reduces the level of functional vitamin K-dependent factors II (prothrombin), VII, IX and X by preventing their γ-carboxylation. Novel oral anticoagulant development has focused on the synthesis of selective inhibitors of coagulation factor, preferably acting independently of cofactors. The novel anticoagulants act on a number of targets in the coagulation cascade, but two of its key factors, Xa and IIa (thrombin), appear to be particularly promising. As they are involved in the final steps of the coagulation cascade, their inhibition allows blocking of both intrinsic (plasma) and extrinsic (tissue) coagulation pathways.

Because the serine protease thrombin is the final mediator in the coagulation cascade that leads to the production of fibrin, the main protein component of blood clots [1], and is also a potent activator of platelets, it has been a popular target for the development of novel anticoagulants [2]. Several direct thrombin inhibitors (DTIs) have been approved for clinical use in the prevention of thrombosis, for example desirudin. However, these agents still require parenteral administration, limiting their chronic use, and the need for development of efficient, safe, convenient and predictable oral anticoagulants remains.

Historical excursus: ximelagatran

Ximelagatran, a prodrug of melagatran, was the first oral DTI used in clinical trials from 1999. Its reproducible pharmacokinetic characteristics, rapid onset of action and relatively few interactions with food and other drugs raised hopes that it would allow effective oral anticoagulation without the need for regular international normalised ratio (INR) monitoring. Advanced phase III clinical trials proved ximelagatran to be a potent anticoagulant with ability to prevent venous thromboembolism (VTE) at least as efficiently as injections of the low molecular weight heparin (LMWH) enoxaparin followed by administration of warfarin [3]. Ximelagatran has also been found to be safe treatment in terms of risk of haemorrhage. However, the randomised, double-blind, Thrombin Inhibitor in Venous Thromboembolism Treatment (THRIVE) trial and further studies revealed that treatment with ximelagatran carried substantial risk of hepatotoxicity [4]. On the basis of health concerns ximelagatran did not receive FDA approval and it was subsequently withdrawn by AstraZeneca following the EXTEND study because of fear of liver toxicity [5]. The EXTEND study was terminated due to a case of severe acute liver injury just 3 weeks after completion of the 35-day course of treatment.

Dabigatran etexilate

Dabigatran is a potent non-peptide DTI, but it is not orally active and so its physicochemical characteristics were modified to produce a prodrug, dabigatran etexilate (Boehringer Ingelheim Corp.; Figure 5.1). This differs from dabigatran by an ethyl group at the carboxylic acid and a hexyloxycarbonyl side chain at the amidine, and it has strong and long-lasting anticoagulant effects after oral administration [6]. Dabigatran etexilate possesses a number of qualities that make it potentially an attractive and promising novel anticoagulant. It has rapid absorption (onset of action within 2 hours) and its half-life is about 8 hours after single-dose administration and up to 14–17 hours after multiple doses (Figure 5.2) [7].

Dabigatran etexilate is a double prodrug that is converted by esterases into its active metabolite, dabigatran, once it has been absorbed from the gastrointestinal tract. As bioconversion of dabigatran etexilate to dabigatran begins in the gut, the drug enters the portal vein as a combination of pro-drug and active compound.

Dabigatran etexilate

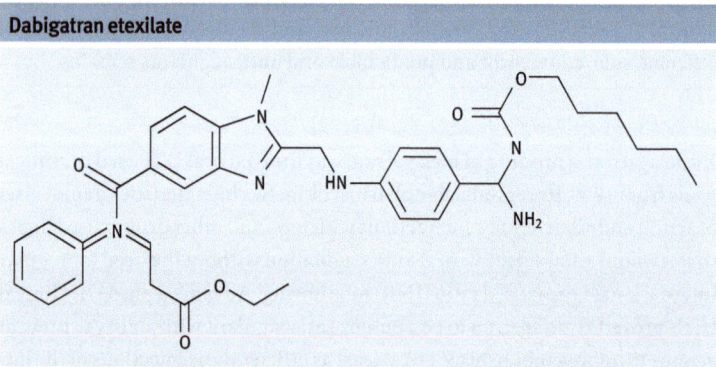

Figure 5.1 Dabigatran etexilate.

Properties of dabigatran etexilate, rivaroxaban and apixaban			
	Dabigatran etexilate	**Rivaroxaban**	**Apixaban**
Target	Thrombin	Factor Xa	Factor Xa
Prodrug	Yes	No	No
Bioavailability (%)	6.5	>80	>50
Time to peak level (h)	2–3	2–4	3
Half-life (h)	14–17	9	9–14
Renal excretion (%)	80	33 (67% by liver)	25 (~70% in faeces)
Dosing	Once or twice daily	Once or twice daily	Once or twice daily
Drug interactions	Potent CYP3A4 and P-glycoprotein inhibitors	Potent CYP3A4 and P-glycoprotein inhibitors	Proton pump inhibitors
Antidote	No	No	No

Figure 5.2 Properties of dabigatran etexilate, rivaroxaban and apixaban.

The cytochrome P450 system plays no part in the metabolism of dabigatran etexilate. Therefore, the risk of drug interactions is low. Because the bioavailability of dabigatran etexilate is only 6.5%, relatively high doses of the drug must be given to ensure that adequate plasma concentrations are achieved. The absorption of dabigatran etexilate in the stomach and small intestine is dependent on an acid environment. To promote such a microenvironment, dabigatran etexilate is provided in tartaric acid-containing capsules. Absorption is reduced by 20–25% if patients are concurrently on proton pump inhibitors [8]. Once it reaches the liver, bioconversion of the pro-drug is completed, and about 20% is conjugated and excreted via the biliary system. About 80% of circulated dabigatran is excreted unchanged via the kidneys. Consequently, plasma concentrations increase in patients with renal insufficiency. It is contraindicated in patients with severe renal failure.

It is noteworthy that dabigatran etexilate has no known interactions with food, as well as having a low potential for drug interactions [2]. Accumulated evidence from completed and ongoing trials confirms the hepatic safety of the drug [9].

In March 2008, the European Commission granted marketing authorisation for dabigatran etexilate (Pradaxa) for the prevention of VTE in adults who have undergone total hip replacement (THR) or total knee replacement (TKR). The drug was launched in the UK in April 2008.

VTE prevention in major joint surgery

Clinical evaluation of dabigatran etexilate started in the setting of major joint surgery. In the multicentre, open-label phase II BISTRO I trial [10], 314 patients undergoing THR were assigned to receive different doses of dabigatran etexilate (12.5, 25, 50, 100, 150, 200 or 300 mg twice daily, or 150 or 300 mg once daily) administered 4–8 hours after surgery for 6–10 days. No major haemorrhages were observed in any group. However, non-major multiple-site haemorrhage was observed in two patients with reduced renal clearance treated with the highest dose (300 mg twice daily). The overall incidence of DVT was 12.4%, without a consistent relationship between incidence and dose. The lowest dose (12.5 mg twice daily) showed a high rate of proximal DVT (12.5%).

In the subsequent phase II BISTRO II trial [11] the 1973 patients undergoing THR or TKR were randomised to 6–10 days of dabigatran etexilate (50, 150 or 225 mg twice daily, or 300 mg once daily) starting 1–4 hours after surgery, or enoxaparin (40 mg once daily) starting 12 hours prior to surgery. VTE occurred in 28.5, 17.4, 13.1, 16.6 and 24% of patients assigned to dabigatran etexilate 50, 150, 225 mg twice daily, 300 mg once daily and enoxaparin, respectively. Compared with enoxaparin, VTE was significantly lower in patients receiving 150 or 225 mg twice daily or 300 mg once daily, and major haemorrhage was significantly lower with 50 mg twice daily but elevated with higher doses, nearly achieving statistical significance with the 300 mg once daily dose ($p = 0.051$). Together, the BISTRO I and BISTRO II trials showed that dabigatran etexilate might be an effective and safe anticoagulant and served as a basis for dose justification in phase III trials.

The clinical utility of dabigatran etexilate for the prevention of VTE in patients after major joint surgery was confirmed in two large randomised, double-blind, multi-centre, placebo-controlled trials (Figure 5.3). The RE-MODEL trial [12] compared dabigatran etexilate (150 mg or 220 mg once daily, starting with a half-dose 1–4 hours after TKR) and enoxaparin (40 mg once daily starting the evening before surgery in 2,076 patients). The treatment continued for 6–10 days and patients were followed up for 3 months. The primary efficacy outcome of a composite of total VTE (venographic or symptomatic) and mortality during treatment occurred in 37.7% of patients in the enoxaparin group, 36.4% of the dabigatran etexilate 220 mg group and 40.5% of the 150 mg dabigatran etexilate group. Both dabigatran etexilate doses proved to be non-inferior to enoxaparin. The incidence of major haemorrhage also did not differ significantly across the three groups (1.3, 1.5 and 1.3%, respectively).

A similar design was used in the RE-NOVATE trial [13] to test potential non-inferiority of dabigatran etexilate for VTE prophylaxis in 3,494 patients undergoing THR, except that the treatment was continued for 28–35 days. The primary efficacy outcome, a composite of total VTE and all-cause mortality during treatment, occurred in 6.7% of individuals in the enoxaparin group, 6.0% of patients in the dabigatran etexilate 220 mg group and 8.6% of patients in the 150 mg group, i.e. both the dabigatran etexilate doses were non-inferior to enoxaparin. There was no significant difference in major haemorrhage rates with either dose of dabigatran etexilate compared with enoxaparin. In the ongoing phase III RE-NOVATE II trial (NCT00657150) 1,920 patients scheduled to undergo THR are to be randomised to dabigatran etexilate

Efficacy and safety of dabigatran etexilate in major joint surgery					
	Duration of treatment	Initiation of dabigatran etexilate	Treatment tested	VTE and all-cause mortality (%)	Major haemorrhage (%)
RE-NOVATE (THA) n=3494	6–10 days	1–4 hours post operation (with half dose)	Dabigatran etexilate 150 mg od	6.7	
			Dabigatran etexilate 220 mg od	8.6	
			Enoxaparin 40 mg od	6.0	
RE-MODEL (TKA) n=2076	6–10 days	1–4 hours post operation (with half dose)	Dabigatran etexilate 150 mg od	37.7	
			Dabigatran etexilate 220 mg od	40.5	
			Enoxaparin 40 mg od	36.4	
RE-MOBILIZE (TKA) n=1896	12–15 days	6–12 hours post operation	Dabigatran etexilate 150 mg od	25.3	
			Dabigatran etexilate 220 mg od	33.7*	
			Enoxaparin 30 mg bid	31.1*	

Figure 5.3 Efficacy and safety of dabigatran etexilate in major joint surgery. Bid, twice daily; od, once daily; THA, Total hip arthroplasty; TKA, total knee arthroplasty. *Inferior to enoxaparin.

capsules (110 mg administered on the day of surgery followed by 220 mg once daily) or enoxaparin 40 mg once daily for 28–35 days.

No significant differences in the incidences of liver enzyme elevation and acute coronary events were observed during treatment or follow-up in the RE-MODEL and the RE-NOVATE trials.

The successful record of dabigatran etexilate in preceding clinical trials was partly compromised in the double-blind, centrally randomised RE-MOBILIZE trial [14], in which the North American recommended dose for VTE prophylaxis was used for the enoxaparin comparator, (i.e. 30 mg twice daily rather than

40 mg once daily). Dabigatran etexilate 220 or 150 mg once daily was compared with enoxaparin 30 mg twice daily after knee arthroplasty surgery. Among 1,896 patients, dabigatran etexilate at both doses showed inferior efficacy to enoxaparin, with VTE rates of 31% for 220 mg ($p = 0.02$ vs. enoxaparin), 34% for 150 mg ($p < 0.001$ vs. enoxaparin) and 25% for enoxaparin. Major haemorrhage was uncommon in all groups: 0.6% for dabigatran 220 mg, 0.6% for dabigatran 150 mg and 1.4% for enoxaparin (no significant differences). Serious adverse events occurred in 6.9% of dabigatran 220 mg patients, 6.5% of dabigatran 150 mg patients and 5.2% of enoxaparin patients.

An interesting clinical difference between European and North American prophylactic dosing regimens for antithrombotic drugs for perioperative orthopaedic patients is that, historically, European dosing regimens administered these drugs before surgery, whereas in North America dosing began postoperatively, sometimes at a higher total daily dosage [15]. Because dabigatran was first investigated in European joint arthroplasty patients, the LMWH control therapy, enoxaparin, was initiated the evening before the day of surgery at the standard dosage of 40 mg once daily in the phase II studies.

VTE treatment

The promising efficacy results for dabigatran in the prevention of thromboembolic disorders prompted the developers to test the drug's utility in VTE treatment (Figure 5.4). There are three ongoing trials.

In the phase III, randomised, non-inferiority RE-COVER study (NCT00291330 [2,564 participants]) and in NCT00680186 (2,554 patients) patients with acute symptomatic VTE are to be randomised for 6 months of 150 mg twice daily dabigatran etexilate or warfarin following initial (5–10 days) parenteral anticoagulation. The efficacy and safety of dabigatran etexilate for 6 months will be evaluated, the primary endpoint being a composite of recurrent symptomatic VTE (DVT or PE) and death related to VTE. Recruitment for these studies has been completed and the results are awaited in the near future.

In a separate phase III randomised multicentre trial (NCT00558259) the efficacy of prolonged (additional 12 months) administration of dabigatran etexilate in 1,547 patients with VTE will be compared with placebo. Additionally, the RE-MEDY (NCT00329238) trial aims to evaluate the comparative safety and efficacy of dabigatran etexilate and warfarin for the long-term treatment and secondary prevention of symptomatic VTE in patients who have already been successfully treated with a standard anticoagulant approach for 3–6 months for confirmed acute symptomatic VTE. The planned duration of the treatment is 18 months, and 2,500 patients are to be recruited.

Clinical development programme for dabigatran etexilate		
Clinical condition	**Trial**	**Comparator (n)**
VTE prevention in major joint surgery	Phase II BISTRO I	No comparator (314)
	BISTRO II	Enoxaparin (1,973)
	Phase III RE-MODEL (NCT00168805)	Enoxaparin (2,076)
	RE-NOVATE (NCT00168818)	Enoxaparin (3,494)
	RE-MOBILIZE	Enoxaparin (1,896)
	RE-NOVATE II (NCT00657150)	Enoxaparin (1,920)
VTE treatment	Phase III RE-COVER (NCT00291330)	Parenteral anticoagulant/warfain (2,564)
	NCT00680186	Parenteral anticoagulant/warfarin (2,554)
	NCT00558259	Placebo (1,547)
	RE-MEDY (NCT00329238)	Warfarin (2,500)
Stroke prevention in atrial fibrillation	Phase II PETRO	Aspirin or warfarin (502)
	Phase III RE-LY (NCT00262600)	Warfarin (18,000)
	RELY-ABLE (NCT00808067)	Placebo (6,200)
Acute coronary syndrome	RE-DEEM (NCT0062185)	Placebo (1,878)
Percutaneous coronary intervention	NCT00818753	Heparin (50)

Figure 5.4 Clinical development programme for dabigatran etexilate. VTE, venous thromboembolism.

Stroke prevention in atrial fibrillation

The clinical safety of dabigatran etexilate (with or without aspirin) in patients with AF was first assessed in the phase II dose-range PETRO trial [16]. 502 patients with AF were randomised to receive 50, 150 or 300 mg twice daily of dabigatran etexilate alone or combined with 81 or 325 mg of aspirin or warfarin for 12 weeks. Major haemorrhage was limited to the group treated with 300 mg dabigatran plus aspirin (4 of 64), and the incidence was significant versus 300 mg dabigatran alone (0 of 105, p <0.02). Total haemorrhage events were more frequent in the 300 mg (23%) and 150 mg (18%) dabigatran groups compared with the 50 mg groups (7%; $p = 0.0002$ and $p = 0.01$, respectively). The study demonstrated that major haemorrhages were limited to patients treated with dabigatran 300 mg plus aspirin, and thromboembolic episodes were limited to the 50 mg dabigatran groups. On the basis of the PETRO study 150 and 220 mg doses were chosen for further development in phase III studies of stroke prevention in AF.

The Randomized Evaluation of Long term anticoagulant therapy (RE-LY) with dabigatran etexilate trial (NCT00262600) recently compared the efficacy and safety of two doses of dabigatran etexilate with warfarin in over 18,000 patients with AF with an average age of 71 years. The primary outcome measure was the incidence of stroke (including hemorrhagic) and systemic embolism at the median 2-year follow-up period. Treatment with the higher, 150-mg twice daily dose significantly reduced stroke risk (with a relative risk of 0.66; p <0.001, the rate of hemorrhagic stroke was 0.38% per year in the warfarin group vs 0.10% per year with dabigatran, p <0.001), with a similar overall risk to warfarin for major bleeding. The lower, 110-mg dose resulted in a similar risk for stroke as warfarin but with a significantly reduced major bleeding event rate (20% relative risk reduction, 3.36% per year in the warfarin group vs 2.71% per year with dabigatran, p = 0.003). The rate of haemorrhagic stroke was 0.38% per year in the warfarin group, as compared with 0.12% per year with 110 mg dabigatran (p <0.001) and 0.10% per year with 150 mg of dabigatran (p <0.001). Annual mortality rate was 4.13% in the warfarin group, 3.75% with 110 mg of dabigatran and 3.64% with 150 mg of dabigatran (borderline significance, p = 0.051) [17] (Figure 5.5). The second trial, RELY-ABLE, is investigating the safety of more prolonged treatment with dabigatran etexilate in those who completed the RE-LY trial, with the recruitment target of 6,200 patients.

Other directions

The potential application of DTIs is not limited by conditions related to venous thrombosis, and dabigatran etexilate is also being tested in phase II trials in clinical settings of arterial thrombosis. In the Randomized, Open Label Study of Dabigatran Etexilate in Elective Percutaneous Coronary Intervention (NCT00818753) two doses of dabigatran etexilate (110 and 150 mg twice daily) are being compared with heparin (both in addition to a standard dual antiplatelet regimen) in 50 patients undergoing elective percutaneous coronary intervention (PCI). A larger (n = 1,878) placebo-controlled trial, Dose Finding Study for Dabigatran Etexilate in Patients With Acute Coronary Syndrome (RE-DEEM; NCT00621855), is evaluating the safety and potential of efficacy of four different dabigatran doses administered twice daily for 6 months in addition to dual antiplatelet treatment in patients with acute coronary syndrome (ACS) with high risk of cardiovascular complications.

Additionally, the safety and tolerability of dabigatran etexilate are now being evaluated in adolescent patients with VTE (phase II trial NCT00844415), and a

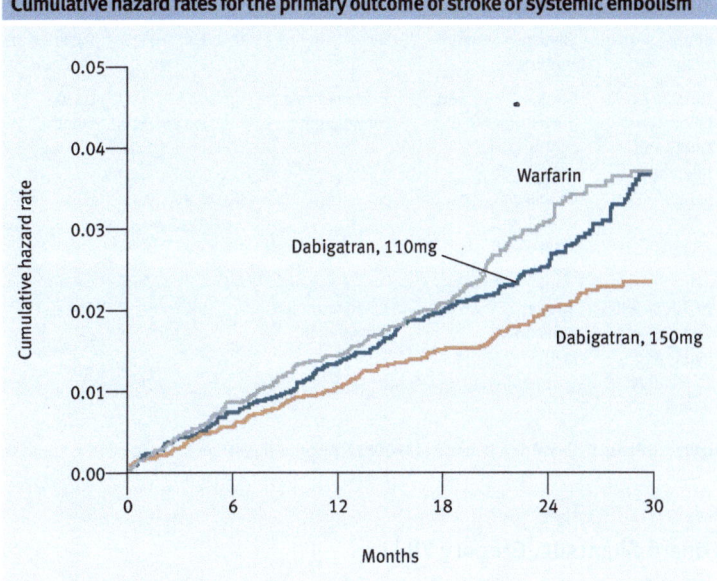

Cumulative hazard rates for the primary outcome of stroke or systemic embolism

Figure 5.5 Cumulative hazard rates for the primary outcome of stroke or systemic embolism, according to treatment group. Reproduced with permission from Connolly SJ et al. [17].

number of ongoing observational cohort studies aim to further optimise clinical management with dabigatran (NCT00846807, NCT00847301) by selection of specific patient groups (e.g. with moderate renal impairment) and treatment regimes.

AZD0837

AZD0837 is a novel oral DTI that is under development by Astra-Zeneca for potential treatment of thrombosis and prevention of thromboembolism in AF (Figure 5.6). Clinical data from phase II trials on AZD0837 150 mg twice daily revealed that it has a low and predictable incidence of increased liver alanine transaminase (ALT), comparable to warfarin. The extended-release formulation ensures no peak and troughs over 24 hours. There is also minimal interaction with other drugs and no food interaction, as well as less frequent haemorrhage than with warfarin. AZD0837 has active/intermediate metabolites, AR-H067637XX and AR-H069927XX, and the main route of secretion appears to be biliary.

Phase II clinical development of AZD0837					
Study	Clinical condition	n	Dose	Control	Duration of treatment
NCT00623779 (short-term safety and tolerability study)	Stroke prevention in AF in those unable or unwilling to take VKA therapy	150	Extended-release formulation	VKA antagonists	Up to 3 months
NCT00645853 (long-term safety and tolerability study)	Stroke prevention in AF	523	Extended-release formulation	VKA antagonists	5 years

Figure 5.6 Phase II clinical development of AZD0837. AF, atrial fibrillation; VKA, vitamin K antagonist.

Factor Xa inhibitors
Eduard Shantsila, Gregory YH Lip

Factor Xa represents an attractive target for antithrombotic drugs. Blockade of factor Xa permits inhibition of both the extrinsic and intrinsic coagulation pathways and has promise in the effective management of thrombotic disorders, though admittedly their clinical utility of factor Xa inhibitors will depend on their safety and on whether they have predictable pharmacokinetics. Several factor Xa inhibitors are currently in clinical development, rivaroxaban and apixaban being in the most advanced stages. A number of other factor Xa inhibitors, such as betrixaban (PRT-054021), DU-176b (edoxaban), YM150 and LY517717, are also in clinical studies (Figure 5.7).

Clinical development of the novel factor Xa inhibitors			
Clinical condition	Phase	Trial title	Comparator (n)
Betrixaban [PRT054021] (Portola Pharmaceuticals)			
VTE prevention in major joint surgery	II	Factor Xa Inhibitor, PRT054021, Against Enoxaparin for the Prevention of Venous Thromboembolic Events (EXPERT) [NCT00375609]	Enoxaparin (200)
Stroke prevention in atrial fibrillation	II	Study of the Safety, Tolerability and Pilot Efficacy of Oral Factor Xa Inhibitor Betrixaban Compared to Warfarin (EXPLORE-Xa) [NCT00742859]	Warfarin (500)

Figure 5.7 Clinical development of the novel factor Xa inhibitors. VTE, venous thromboembolism. Continued opposite.

Clinical development of the novel factor Xa inhibitors

DU-176b (Daiichi Sankyo Inc.)

VTE prevention in major joint surgery	II	A Study of DU-176b in Preventing Blood Clots After Hip Replacement Surgery [NCT00107900]	Not specified in (402)
	II	Study of the Efficacy and Safety of DU-176b in Preventing Blood Clots in Patients Undergoing Total Hip Replacement [NCT00398216]	Dalteparin (950)
Stroke prevention in atrial fibrillation		A Study to Assess the Safety of a Potential New Drug in Comparison to the Standard Practice of Dosing With Warfarin for Non-Valvular Atrial Fibrillation [NCT00504556]	Warfarin (2,000)
	II	DU-176b Phase 2 Dose Finding Study in Subjects With Non-Valvular Atrial Fibrillation [NCT00806624]	Warfarin (235)
	II	Late Phase 2 Study of DU-176b in Patients With Non-Valvular Atrial Fibrillation [NCT00829933]	Warfarin (536)
	III	Global Study to Assess the Safety and Effectiveness of DU-176b vs Standard Practice of Dosing With Warfarin in Patients With Atrial Fibrillation (EngageAFTIMI48) [NCT00781391]	Warfarin (16,500)

YM150 (Astellas Pharma Inc.)

VTE prevention in major joint surgery	II	A Study to Evaluate the Safety and Efficacy of YM150 in Patients With Knee Replacement (PEARL) [NCT00595426]	Warfarin (625)
	II	Factor Xa Inhibitor for Prevention of Venous Thromboembolism in Patients Undergoing Elective Total Knee Replacement (PEARL-1) [NCT00408239]	Enoxaparin (367)
	II	Factor Xa Inhibitor YM150 for the Prevention of Blood Clot Formation in Veins After Scheduled Hip Replacement (ONYX-2) [NCT00353678]	Enoxaparin (1139)
	II	A Study Evaluating Efficacy and Safety of YM150 Compared to Enoxaparin in Subjects Undergoing Hip Replacement Surgery (ONYX-3) [NCT00902928]	Enoxaparin (2,000)

Figure 5.7 Clinical development of the novel factor Xa inhibitors. VTE, venous thromboembolism. Continued overleaf.

Clinical development of the novel factor Xa inhibitors

Stroke prevention in atrial fibrillation	II	Direct Factor Xa Inhibitor YM150 for Prevention of Stroke in Subjects With Non-Valvular Atrial Fibrillation [NCT00448214]	Warfarin (448)
LY517717 (Eli Lilly)			
VTE prevention in major joint surgery	II	New Oral Anticoagulant Therapy for the Prevention of Blood Clots Following Hip or Knee Replacement Surgery [NCT00074828]	Enoxaparin (511)
TAK-442 (Takeda Global Research & Development Center, Inc.)			
VTE prevention in major joint surgery	II	Efficacy and Safety of TAK-442 in Subjects Undergoing Total Knee Replacement [NCT00641732]	Enoxaparin (1,045)
Otamixaban/XRP0673 (Sanofi-Aventis)			
Percutaneous coronary intervention	II	The SEPIA-PCI Trial: Otamixaban in Comparison to Heparin in Subjects Undergoing Non-Urgent Percutaneous Coronary Intervention [NCT00133731]	Unfractionated heparin (947)
Non-ST elevation Acute coronary syndrome	II	Study of Otamixaban Versus Unfractionated Heparin (UFH) and Eptifibatide in Non-ST Elevation Acute Coronary Syndrome (SEPIA-ACS1) [NCT00317395]	Unfractionated heparin, eptifibatide (3,240)

Figure 5.7 Clinical development of the novel factor Xa inhibitors.

Rivaroxaban

Rivaroxaban (Bayer Healthcare AG; Figure 5.8) is a novel factor Xa inhibitor that exhibits predictable pharmacokinetics, with high oral bioavailability, rapid onset of action (achieves maximum plasma concentration in 1.5–2.0 hours) and no known food interactions [18]. The drug has a dual mode of elimination: two-thirds of it is metabolised by the liver (mostly via CYP3A4 and CYP2J2), with no major or active circulating metabolites identified, and one-third is excreted unchanged by the kidneys. Elimination of rivaroxaban from plasma occurs with a terminal half-life of 5–9 hours in young individuals, and with a terminal half-life of 12–13 hours in subjects aged >75 years [19]. Available data indicate that body weight, age, and gender do not have a clinically relevant effect on the pharmacokinetics and pharmacodynamics of rivaroxaban, and it thus can be administered in fixed doses without coagulation monitoring. Rivaroxaban has minimal drug interactions (eg, with naproxen, acetylsalicylic acid, clopidogrel, or digoxin) [18]. Its predictable pharmacokinetics and pharmacodynamics allow use of rivaroxaban without regular laboratory monitoring. Although no specific antidote is known for rivaroxaban, preclinical data suggest that recombinant factor VIIa and activated prothrombin complex concentrate may reverse the effects of high-dose rivaroxaban.

Rivaroxaban

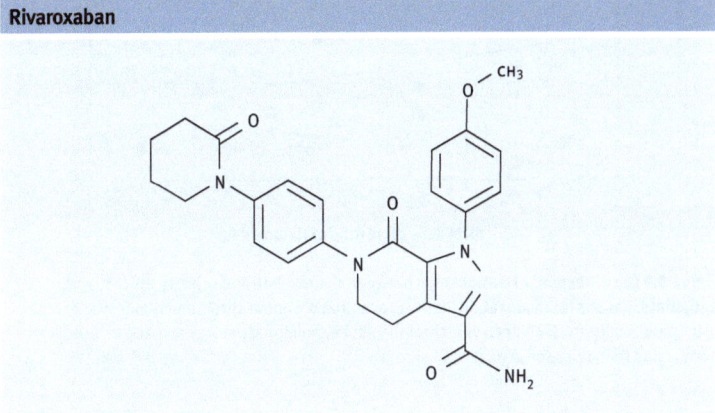

Figure 5.8 Rivaroxaban.

VTE prevention

Four completed phase II efficacy and safety studies of rivaroxaban for the prevention of VTE in patients undergoing elective THR and TKR (n = 2,907 patients) have demonstrated comparable efficacy and safety of rivaroxaban and conventional management with subcutaneous enoxaparin [20–23]. Efficacy was assessed as a composite of any DVT (proximal or distal), non-fatal objectively confirmed PE and all-cause mortality; safety was judged on the basis of major haemorrhage incidence. A pooled analysis of two of these studies confirmed non-inferiority of rivaroxaban in patients undergoing elective THR or TKR, with no significant dose–response relationship for efficacy but with a significant dose-related increase for the primary safety endpoint (p <0.001), a total daily dose of 5–20 mg being the optimal dose range (Figure 5.9) [24].

Consequently, a fixed dose of rivaroxaban 10 mg once daily was selected to be used in the phase III RECORD programme (Figure 5.10). The RECORD

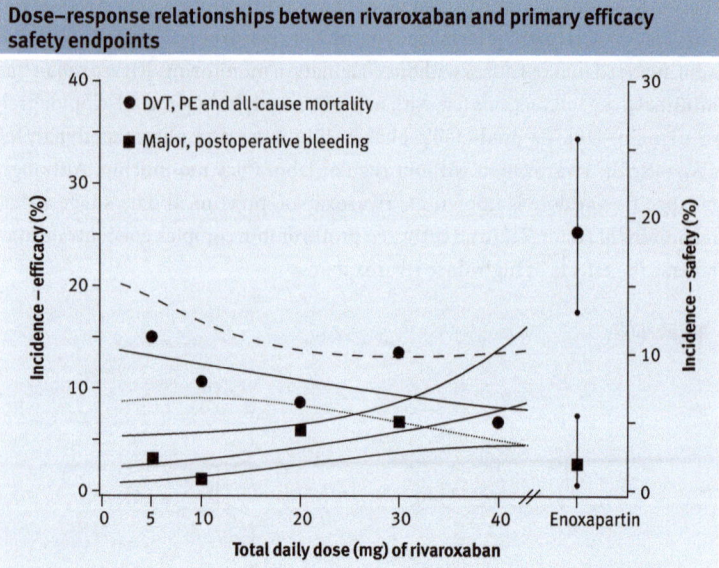

Figure 5.9 Dose–response relationships between rivaroxaban and primary efficacy safety endpoints. Results for rivaroxaban for the prevention of venous thromboembolism after major orthopaedic surgery. DVT, deep vein thrombosis; PE, pulmonary embolism. Reproduced with permission from Eriksson et al. [20].

programme includes four large trials recruiting more than 12,500 patients undergoing elective THR or TKR. All RECORD trials have the primary efficacy endpoint of the composite of DVT, non-fatal PE and all-cause mortality, and the main secondary efficacy endpoint was major VTE. The primary safety endpoint was major haemorrhage. These studies had no upper age limit and allowed recruitment of patients with mild or moderate hepatic impairment.

The RECORD1 and the RECORD3 studies compared rivaroxaban 10 mg once daily (starting 6–8 hours after surgery) with enoxaparin 40 mg once daily (starting the evening before surgery) both given for 31–39 days (extended prophylaxis) after THR (RECORD1) [25] or for 10–14 days (short-term prophylaxis) after TKR (RECORD3) [26]. In both studies treatment with rivaroxaban was significantly superior to enoxaparin for VTE prevention. Recognising that current guidelines recommend extended prophylaxis for patients undergoing THR, although this is not done in many countries, the RECORD2 trial investigated the efficacy and safety of extended thromboprophylaxis with rivaroxaban (5 weeks) compared with short-term enoxaparin 40 mg once daily for 10–14 days [27]. The study demonstrated that prolonged

Incidence of venous thromboembolism and haemorrhage in the RECORD programme.

Trial	Regimen (once daily)	Duration of treatment	Total VTE (%)	p	Major VTE (%)	p	Symptomatic VTE (%)	p	Major haemorrhage (%)	Clinically relevant non-major haemorrhage
RECORD1 (THR) n = 4,541	Rivaroxaban 10 mg	5 weeks	1.1	<0.0001	0.2	<0.0001	0.3	0.22	0.3	2.9
	Enoxaparin 40 mg	5 weeks	3.7		2.0		0.5		0.1	2.4
RECORD2 (THR) n = 2,509	Rivaroxaban 10 mg	10–14 days	2.0	<0.0001	0.6	<0.0001	0.2	0.004	<0.1	3.3
	Enoxaparin 40 mg	5 weeks	9.3		5.1		1.2		<0.1	2.7
RECORD3 (TKR) n = 2,531	Rivaroxaban 10 mg	10–14 days	9.6	<0.001	1.0	0.01	0.7	0.005	0.6	2.7
	Enoxaparin 40 mg	10–14 days	18.9		2.6		2.0		0.5	2.3
RECORD4 (TKR) n = 3,148	Rivaroxaban 10 mg	10–14 days	6.9	0.012	1.2	0.124	0.7	0.187	0.7	NA
	Enoxaparin 40 mg	10–14 days	10.1		2.0		1.2		0.3	NA

Figure 5.10. Incidence of venous thromboembolism (VTE) and haemorrhage in the RECORD programme. NA, not available; THR, total hip replacement; TKR, total knee replacement.

prophylaxis with rivaroxaban was associated with reduced incidence of VTE, including symptomatic events after THR. Of note, despite administration of rivoxaban for 3 weeks longer than enoxaparin, the rate of major haemorrhage at 5 weeks was low and similar in both groups. In the RECORD4 trial [28] rivaroxaban 10 mg was significantly more effective than the North American regimen of enoxaparin 30 mg twice daily (10–14 days) in patients undergoing TKR, with similar rates of major haemorrhage for both treatments and no serious liver toxicity with rivaroxaban. Thus the superiority of rivaroxaban over enoxaparin for VTE prevention was demonstrated in all four studies, with a good safety profile. As a result, rivaroxaban has recently received approval in the European Union and in Canada for the prevention of VTE in patients undergoing elective THR or TKR surgery.

The utility of rivaroxaban (10 mg once daily for up to 5 weeks) for VTE prevention in hospitalised medically ill patients is currently being assessed in a phase III MAGELLAN study, with short-term enoxaparin as the comparator (NCT00571649).

Treatment of VTE

The initial phase IIb ODIXa-DVT [29] and EINSTEIN-DVT [30] studies (Figure 5.11) assessed the clinical efficacy and safety of rivaroxaban for the treatment of VTE in patients with acute, symptomatic, proximal DVT without symptomatic PE. The treatment was prescribed for 3 months, with open-label standard therapy (LMWH/heparin following VKA) as comparator.

In the ODIXa-DVT study [29], rivaroxaban doses 10, 20 or 30 mg twice daily, or 40 mg once daily, were tested. The primary efficacy endpoint of reduced thrombus burden on day 21 (assessed by quantitative compression ultrasonography) without recurrent VTE or VTE-related death was registered in 43.8–59.2% of patients receiving rivaroxaban and in 45.9% of patients receiving standard therapy. The incidence of the primary safety endpoint (major haemorrhage) was 1.7–3.3% in the rivaroxaban groups; there were no events in the standard therapy group.

In the EINSTEIN-DVT study [30], therapy with rivaroxaban 20–40 mg once daily was associated with an incidence of 5.4–6.6% for the primary endpoint (the composite of symptomatic, recurrent VTE and deterioration of thrombotic burden, as assessed by compression ultrasound and perfusion lung scan) compared with 9.9% in the standard therapy group. The primary safety endpoint (any clinically relevant haemorrhage) developed in 2.9–7.5% of patients receiving rivaroxaban and 8.8% of those on the standard therapy, with no evidence of compromised liver function in those receiving rivaroxaban.

The ODIXa-DVT and EINSTEIN-DVT studies

ODIXa-DVT study

	Rivaroxaban				Enoxaparin + VKA
	10 mg bid	20 mg bid	30 mg bid	40 mg bid	
	($n = 100$)	($n = 98$)	($n = 109$)	($n = 112$)	($n = 109$)
Improvement in thrombus burden without recurrent VTE at 3 weeks (%)	53.0	59.2	56.9	43.8	45.9
Recurrent DVT, PE, and VTE-related death at 3 months, n (%)	2 (1.9)	2 (2.0)	2 (1.8)	3 (2.6)	1 (0.9)
Major haemorrhage, n (%)	2 (1.7)	2 (1.7)	4 (3.3)	2 (1.7)	0

EINSTEIN-DVT study

	Rivaroxaban			LMWH/ heparin + VKA
	20 mg od	30 mg od	40 mg od	
	($n = 115$)	($n = 112$)	($n = 121$)	($n = 101$)
Recurrent VTE and thrombus deterioration at 3 months, n (%)	7 (6.1)	6 (5.4)	8 (6.6)	10 (9.9)
Major haemorrhage, n (%)	1 (0.7)	2 (1.5)	0 (0.0)	2 (1.5)

Figure 5.11 The ODIXa-DVT and EINSTEIN-DVT studies. DVT, deep vein thrombosis; LMWH, low-molecular-weight heparin; od, once daily; PE, pulmonary embolism; VKA, vitamin K antagonist; VTE, venous thromboembolism.

Of note, the phase II studies revealed that the twice-daily rivaroxaban regimen was more effective for thrombus regression at 3 weeks, whereas the once- and twice-daily regimens showed similar effectiveness at 3-month follow-up [29]. Accordingly, an initial intensified twice-daily regimen (rivaroxaban 15 mg twice daily for 3 weeks) followed by long-term 20 mg once daily dosing was chosen for investigation in the ongoing phase III EINSTEIN studies: EINSTEIN-DVT (NCT00440193), EINSTEIN-PE (NCT00439777) and EINSTEIN-EXTENSION (NCT00439725).

The multicentre, randomised, open-label EINSTEIN-DVT and EINSTEIN-PE studies (Figure 5.12) are investigating the efficacy and safety of rivaroxaban in patients with confirmed symptomatic DVT or PE in comparison to enoxaparin, followed by a VKA (standard therapy) for a predefined treatment period of 3, 6 or 12 months. The EINSTEIN-EXTENSION study is now recruiting patients who have been treated for 6 or 12 months with rivaroxaban or a VKA to receive rivaroxaban 20 mg once daily or placebo for a further 6 or 12 months.

Ongoing phase III clinical development programme for rivaroxaban.		
Clinical condition	**Trial**	**Comparator**
VTE prevention in medically ill patients	MAGELLAN (NCT00571649)	Standard enoxaparin therapy
Stroke prevention in atrial fibrillation	ROCKET AF (NCT00403767) J-ROCKET (NCT00494871)	Standard warfarin therapy
Secondary prevention of cardiovascular events in acute coronary syndrome	ATLAS 2 TIMI 51 (NCT00809965)	Placebo, in addition to standard therapy
VTE treatment	EINSTEIN- DVT (NCT00440193) EINSTEIN-PE (NCT00439777) EINSTEIN-EXTENSION (NCT00439725)	Vitamin K antagonists

Figure 5.12 Ongoing phase III clinical development programme for rivaroxaban. VTE, venous thromboembolism.

Stroke prevention in atrial fibrillation

In terms of numbers of patients, stroke prevention in AF is potentially the largest category that may benefit from the novel oral anticoagulants. The rising incidence of AF in a progressively ageing population suggests that millions of people may eventually require life-long anticoagulant therapy to prevent severely disabling complications. To assess the utility of rivaroxaban for AF the Embolism Trial in Atrial Fibrillation (ROCKET AF) study is investigating the effectiveness and safety of rivaroxaban 20 mg once daily (15 mg once daily in those with moderate kidney impairment) versus warfarin for the prevention of stroke in about 14,000 patients with AF (NCT00403767). In the J-ROCKET AF study being conducted in Japan, lower doses of rivaroxaban 10 mg once daily (5 mg once daily for patients with moderate renal impairment) are to be compared with warfarin (NCT00494871).

Acute coronary syndromes

Preclinical data indicated the possible effectiveness of rivaroxaban and other factor Xa inhibitors and DTIs in clinical settings of arterial thrombosis. In the phase IIb Anti-Xa Therapy to Lower cardiovascular events in Addition to aspirin with/without thienopyridine therapy in Subjects with Acute Coronary Syndrome [ATLAS ACS (TIMI 46)] study, about 3,500 patients with recent ACS were randomised to escalating total daily doses of rivaroxaban, ranging from 5 mg up to 20 mg (once or twice daily), or placebo, in addition to the standard antiplatelet therapy of aspirin or aspirin plus a thienopyridine (eg, clopidogrel) for secondary prevention of cardiovascular events. Patients on the rivaroxaban regimens had higher rates of haemorrhage than those on placebo, and the risk increased in a dose-dependent manner; however, no study arm was stopped due to increased haemorrhage. A strong trend towards reduction in cardiovascular events was observed with rivaroxaban, which reduced the main secondary efficacy endpoint of death, myocardial infarction or stroke compared with placebo ($p = 0.0270$) [31]. Two doses of rivaroxaban, 2.5 and 5 mg twice daily, have been chosen for a phase III ATLAS 2 TIMI 51 study, which aims to recruit approximately 16,000 patients with ACS (Figure 5.12).

Apixaban

Apixaban (Bristol-Myers Squibb Co and Pfizer Inc.; Figure 5.13) is another potent, highly selective and reversible inhibitor of factor X and is active against both free enzyme and factor X bound within the prothrombinase complex. The bioavailability of apixaban after oral absorption is over 50% [32]. Peak plasma levels of apixaban are observed 3 hours after administration and plasma concentrations reach the steady state by day 3. The half-life of apixaban is between 8 and 15 hours, which allows once- or twice-daily administration of the drug. The primary elimination route is faecal, with only about 25%

Clinical development of apixaban

Clinical condition	Trial	Comparator
Total knee replacement	ADVANCE-1 (NCT00371683) ADVANCE-2 [NCT00452530)	Enoxaparin
Total hip replacement	ADVANCE-3 (NCT00423319)	Enoxaparin
Stroke prevention in atrial fibrillation	AVERROES (NCT00496769) ARISTOTLE (NCT00412984)	Aspirin Warfarin
Thromboprophylaxis in cancer	ADVOCATE (NCT00320255)	Placebo
Thromboprophylaxis in heart failure, acute respiratory failure or infection (without septic shock), or acute rheumatic disorder or inflammatory bowel disease	ADOPT (NCT00457002)	Enoxaparin
VTE treatment	AMPLIFY (NCT00643201)	Enoxaparin/warfarin
	AMPLIFY-EXT (NCT00633893)	Placebo
Acute coronary syndrome	Phase II APPRAISE-1 (NCT00313300)	Vitamin K antagonists

Figure 5.13 **Clinical development of apixaban.** VTE, venous thromboembolism.

eliminated via the kidney. Apixaban has little effect on the prothrombin time at therapeutic concentrations, but plasma levels can be assessed using a factor Xa inhibition assay.

VTE prevention in major joint surgery

In a randomised phase II dose–response clinical trial (NCT00097357) in 1,238 patients undergoing TKR, apixaban 5, 10 or 20 mg/day (administered as once or twice daily doses) was compared with enoxaparin (30 mg twice daily) and open-label warfarin. Apixaban and enoxaparin were started 12–24 hours after surgery; the warfarin dose was titrated from the evening of the day of surgery. After 10–14 days of the treatment, bilateral venography was performed and patients were further treated at the attending physician's discretion. The primary endpoint, a composite of VTE events plus all-cause mortality at 42-day follow-up, was significantly lower in the compound apixaban group (8.6%) than in the enoxaparin (15.6%, p <0.02) or warfarin (26.6%, p <0.001) groups. The primary endpoint rates for 2.5 mg apixaban twice daily (9.9%) and 5.0 mg once daily (11.3%) were lower than in the enoxaparin (15.6%) and warfarin group (26.6%). The incidence of major haemorrhage in apixaban-treated patients was low and ranged from 0 (2.5 mg twice daily) to 3.3% (20 mg four times daily), with comparable results for once- and twice-daily administration. No major haemorrhage was observed in the enoxaparin and warfarin groups.

The clinical utility of apixaban for VTE prevention after major joint surgery is being investigated in the ongoing phase III ADVANCE programme (Figure 5.13). In two multicentre, randomised, double-blind, active-controlled clinical trials (ADVANCE-1 [NCT00371683] and ADVANCE-2 [NCT00452530]), the safety and efficacy of oral apixaban (2.5 mg twice daily) versus enoxaparin (30 mg twice daily in ADVANCE-1 and 40 mg once daily in ADVANCE-2) for preventing DVT and PE after TKR is to be evaluated in 3,670 patients in each trial. The duration of treatment is 12 days and primary outcome measures are defined as a combination of asymptomatic and symptomatic DVT, non-fatal PE and all-cause mortality. In a similar ongoing ADVANCE-3 trial (NCT00423319), the efficacy and safety of 5-week administration of apixaban (2.5 mg twice daily) in comparison with enoxaparin in the prevention of DVT and PE is being assessed in 4,424 patients after THR. Patients are randomised to receive apixaban plus placebo or enoxaparin plus placebo for 5 weeks. The primary outcome is a combination of asymptomatic and symptomatic DVT, non-fatal PE and all-cause mortality.

Stroke prevention in atrial fibrillation

Two phase III clinical trials are ongoing to assess apixaban for stroke prevention in patients with AF. In the first, AVERROES study, the effectiveness of oral apixaban (5.0 mg twice daily; or 2.5 mg in selected patients) is being compared with aspirin (81–324 mg once daily) for 36 months in the prevention of stroke or systemic embolism in 6,160 patients with permanent or persistent AF who have at least one additional risk factor for stroke but cannot be treated with VKA.

The second phase III trial, the ARISTOTLE study (NCT00412984), aims to investigate whether apixaban (5 mg twice daily) is as effective as warfarin in preventing stroke and systemic embolism in 16,455 patients with AF who have at least one additional risk factor for stroke.

The primary outcome measure in these two trials is the composite outcome of stroke or systemic embolism.

Thromboprophylaxis in other clinical settings

Apixaban is being tested for several unique applications which may expand the use of oral anticoagulation beyond currently established indications. The phase II randomised ADVOCATE study (NCT00320255) has been designed to determine the tolerability, effectiveness and safety of apixaban in prevention of thrombolic events in patients with advanced or metastatic cancer on prescribed chemotherapy for more than 90 days. Twelve-week administration of apixaban (5 mg once daily) or placebo is to be initiated within 6 weeks of starting chemotherapy in an expected 160 patients.

A further phase III randomised trial, ADOPT (NCT00457002), is comparing the safety and efficacy of apixaban with enoxaparin in preventing DVT and PE in 7,502 patients hospitalised with congestive heart failure, acute respiratory failure, infection (without septic shock), acute rheumatic disorder or inflammatory bowel disease. Patients will receive apixaban (2.5 mg twice daily) for 30 days plus placebo for 6–14 days or enoxaparin (40 mg once daily) for 6–14 days then placebo for 30 days. Primary outcome measures are the composite of VTE and VTE-related death, whereas secondary outcome measures include all-cause mortality, major haemorrhage and clinically relevant non-major haemorrhage.

Treatment of venous thrombosis

Investigation of apixaban utility for treatment of patients with VTE started with the phase II Botticelli DVT dose-ranging clinical trial (NCT00252005). In this study 520 patients with symptomatic DVT were randomised to receive apixaban (5 or 10 mg twice daily or 20 mg four times daily) or traditional treatment with LMWH or fondaparinux followed by VKA. After management for 84–91 days, no significant difference was reported between the treatments in the rate of occurrence of the primary outcome, a composite of symptomatic recurrent VTE and asymptomatic deterioration of bilateral compression ultrasound or perfusion lung scan (4.7% for apixaban and 4.2% in control patients) [32]. The primary outcome rates for the tested apixaban doses were 6.0% for 5.0 mg twice daily, 5.6% for 10.0 mg twice daily and 2.6% for 20.0 mg once daily. The principal safety outcome (a composite of major and clinically relevant non-major haemorrhage) developed at a similar rate in the apixaban-treated patients (7.3%) and the control group (7.9%). The principal safety outcome rates for the tested apixaban doses were 8.6% for 5.0 mg twice daily, 4.5% for 10.0 mg twice daily and 7.3% for 20 mg once daily.

The apixaban research programme continues in phase III trials. In the multicentre, randomised AMPLIFY study (NCT00643201) apixaban is being compared with the conventional treatment (enoxaparin/warfarin) in 3,625 patients with DVT. Apixaban starting at 10 mg twice daily for 7 days is followed by a 5 mg twice daily dose for 6 months. The primary outcome measures are the recurrence of VTE events or death; secondary outcome measures include the incidence of haemorrhage. Additionally, the AMPLIFY-EXT trial (NCT00633893) will assess the efficacy and safety of apixaban in preventing VTE recurrence or death in 2,438 patients with clinical diagnosis of DVT or PE who have already completed their standard treatment for DVT or PE. Patients will receive apixaban (2.5 or 5.0 mg twice daily) or placebo for 12 months.

Acute coronary syndrome

The phase II APPRAISE-1 clinical trial (NCT00313300) is evaluating the safety of apixaban in 1,771 patients with recent ACS. Patients were randomised to receive apixaban (2.5 mg twice daily or 10.0 mg once daily) or placebo for 26 weeks. The primary outcome measure is the incidence of major and clinically relevant non-major haemorrhage; the secondary outcome measure is a composite of death, non-fatal myocardial infarction, severe recurrent ischemia and non-hemorrhagic stroke as well as all haemorrhage events. Preliminary data suggest a trend towards a reduction in cardiovascular events with apixaban, but at the cost of increased haemorrhage related to increasing apixaban dose and concomitant clopidogrel use.

Other novel factor Xa inhibitors

The range of oral factor Xa inhibitors that have reached advanced stages of clinical development is progressively increasing, reflecting interest in the high clinical potential of this pharmaceutical group.

Edoxaban

Edoxaban (DU-176b, Daiichi Sankyo) selectively inhibits factor Xa with high affinity (K_i 0.56 nmol/L). In rat models DU-176b was able to inhibit both arterial and venous thrombosis in the same dose range; in contrast, fondaparinux requires 100-fold higher concentrations to inhibit arterial rather than venous thrombosis. Data from animal models suggest that DU-176b may have a wider therapeutic range than UFH, LMWH, and warfarin, with a lower propensity for haemorrhage. DU-176b was also shown to potentiate the effects of the ticlopidine and tissue plasminogen activator in rat thrombosis models, suggesting that a combination therapy comprising DU-176b and either of these agents may be clinically useful [33]. In a phase I study in healthy males, a single 60 mg dose of DU-176b inhibited factor Xa activity, prolonged both the prothrombin time and activated partial thromboplastin time, and reduced in vitro venous and arterial thrombus formation [34]. The anti-factor Xa activity of DU-176b peaks 1.5 hours after administration and lasts for up to 12 hours, with antithrombotic effects persisting for about 5 hours, suggesting that it has potential for once-daily dosing. There are two ongoing phase II dose-finding studies of DU-176b for the prevention of VTE after THR (NCT00107900 and NCT00398216). The DU-176b programme for stroke prevention in AF has now been extended to a phase III trial, with 16,500 patients to be recruited in the ENGAGE AF-TIMI48 study (NCT00781391).

LY517717

LY517717 (Eli Lilly) is a factor Xa inhibitor with an inhibitory rate constant (K_i) for factor Xa of 4.6–6.6 nmol/L and an an oral bioavailability of 25–82%. It is eliminated mainly by the faecal route, with an elimination half-life of about 25 hours in healthy subjects [35]. In a phase II randomised double-blind dose escalation study (NCT00074828) a dosing range of LY517717 25–150 mg once daily versus enoxaparin 40 mg once daily was tested in 511 patients undergoing TKR or THR [35]. The primary efficacy endpoint was the incidence of VTE at the end of treatment (6–10 days), and safety endpoints were the incidences of major and minor haemorrhage at 30 days after treatment initiation. Three lower doses of LY517717 were stopped due to lack of efficacy, and the three higher doses (100 ,

125 and 150 mg) were non-inferior to the enoxaparin (17.1–24.0% vs 22.2% with enoxaparin for the efficacy endpoint). The three higher LY517717 doses were associated with lower incidences of major haemorrhage (0.0–0.9% vs 1.1% with enoxaparin) and minor haemorrhage (0.0–1.0% vs 2.2% with enoxaparin). Gender and creatinine clearance were found to affect LY517717 exposure and may be partly responsible for the reported intra-individual variability of 35%.

YM150

YM150 (Astellas) is another potent direct factor Xa inhibitor with a K_i of 31 nmol/L. Its active metabolite, YM-222714, also has antithrombotic activity in vivo. YM150 demonstrated potent antithrombotic effects in animal models of venous and arterial thrombosis. In a randomised phase IIa study of 174 patients after THR treatment with 3, 10, 30, or 60 mg once daily of YM150 for 7–10 days, there was a significant dose–response relationship in VTE prevention [36]. No major haemorrhage events were reported in any study arm. Phase IIb ONYX-2 (NCT00353678) and ONYX-3 (NCT00902928) studies have been initiated to assess the efficacy and safety of YM150 in patients undergoing THR, and the phase II PEARL programme will evaluate YM150 in patients after TKR. Additionally, YM150 is being investigated for stroke prevention in patients with AF (NCT00448214).

Betrixaban

Betrixaban (PRT-054021; Portola; licensed from Millennium Pharmaceuticals) specifically and reversibly inhibits factor Xa with a K_i of 0.117 nmol/L. It has a bioavailability of 47% and a half-life of 19 hours, and is excreted almost unchanged in bile. Betrixaban has demonstrated antithrombotic activity in animal models and in human blood and is well tolerated in healthy individuals across a wide range of doses. At present, betrixaban is being investigated in phase II trials for VTE prevention in patients after major joint surgery (EXPERT; NCT00375609) and for stroke prevention in patients with AF (EXPLORE-Xa; NCT00742859) [37].

Other warfarin analogues: ATI-5923 (tecarfarin)
Kok Hoon Tay, Gregory YH Lip

Despite numerous limitations warfarin is a very effective anticoagulant, and attempts are being made to create warfarin analogues that have similar efficacy but also have predictable pharmacodynamics and a convenient scheme of administration, without a need for burdensome monitoring. A novel warfarin analogue, tecarfarin, which is not metabolised by the CYP450 pathway, is currently being tested in the quest for warfarin replacement.

Tecarfarin (ATI-5923), a novel selective inhibitor of the vitamin K epoxide reductase (VKOR inhibitor) developed by ARYx Therapeutics Inc. (Fremont, CA, USA), is not metabolised by the CYP450 pathway. Bypassing CYP450 avoids the numerous drug interactions of warfarin. As a result, more predictable pharmacokinetics and pharmacodynamics are expected. Unlike warfarin, tecarfarin is designed to be metabolised by the esterase pathway; however, it is similar to warfarin in that it inhibits vitamin K dependent coagulation factors (II, VII, IX and X), and hence is a potential anticoagulant for the clinical settings of AF, VTE and mechanical heart valve implantation.

Tecarfarin is currently being studied in the ongoing phase II/III multicentre Embrace-AC study (A Randomized, Double Blind Comparison of ATI-5923, a Novel Vitamin K Antagonist, With Warfarin in Patients Requiring Chronic Anticoagulation [NCT00691470]) to test its superiority against warfarin in maintenance of therapeutic INR ranges in various conditions requiring long-term anticoagulant therapy: atrial flutter/fibrillation, implantation of mechanical heart valves, VTE, history of myocardial infarction or cardiomyopathy requiring oral anticoagulation.

References

1. Mackman N. Triggers, targets and treatments for thrombosis. Nature 2008;451:914–8.
2. Di Nisio M, Middeldorp S, Büller HR. Direct thrombin inhibitors. N Engl J Med 2005;353:1028–40.
3. Wallentin L, Wilcox RG, Weaver WD, et al.; ESTEEM Investigators. Oral ximelagatran for secondary prophylaxis after myocardial infarction: the ESTEEM randomised controlled trial. Lancet 2003;362:789–97.
4. Fiessinger JN, Huisman MV, Davidson BL, et al.; THRIVE Treatment Study Investigators. Ximelagatran vs low-molecular-weight heparin and warfarin for the treatment of deep vein thrombosis: a randomized trial. JAMA 2005;293:681–9.
5. Agnelli G, Eriksson BI, Cohen AT, et al.; on behalf of the EXTEND Study Group. Safety assessment of new antithrombotic agents: Lessons from the EXTEND study on ximelagatran. Thromb Res 2009;123:488–97.
6. Wienen W, Stassen JM, Priepke H, et al. Effects of the direct thrombin inhibitor dabigatran and its orally active prodrug, dabigatran etexilate, on thrombus formation and bleeding time in rats. Thromb Haemost 2007;98:333–8.
7. Stangier J, Stahle H, Rathgen K, Fuhr R. Pharmacokinetics and pharmacodynamics of the direct oral thrombin inhibitor dabigatran in healthy elderly subjects. Clin Pharmacokinet 2008;47:47–59.
8. Stangier J, Rathgen K, Stahle H, et al. The pharmacokinetics, pharmacodynamics and tolerability of dabigatran etexilate, a new oral direct thrombin inhibitor, in healthy male subjects. Br J Clin Pharmacol 2007;64:292–303.
9. Gross PL, Weitz JI. New anticoagulants for treatment of venous thromboembolism. Arterioscler Thromb Vasc Biol 2008;28:380–6.
10. Eriksson BI, Dahl OE, Ahnfelt L, et al. Dose escalating safety study of a new oral direct thrombin inhibitor, dabigatran etexilate, in patients undergoing total hip replacement: BISTRO I. J Thromb Haemost 2004;2:1573–80.
11. Eriksson BI, Dahl OE, Büller HR, et al.; BISTRO II Study Group. A new oral direct thrombin inhibitor, dabigatran etexilate, compared with enoxaparin for prevention of thromboembolic events following total hip or knee replacement: the BISTRO II randomized trial. J Thromb Haemost 2005;3:103–11.
12. Eriksson BI, Dahl OE, Rosencher N, et al.; RE-MODEL Study Group. Oral dabigatran etexilate vs. subcutaneous enoxaparin for the prevention of venous thromboembolism after total knee replacement: the RE-MODEL randomized trial. J Thromb Haemost 2007;5:2178–85.
13. Eriksson BI, Dahl OE, Rosencher N, et al.; RE-NOVATE Study Group. Dabigatran etexilate versus enoxaparin for prevention of venous thromboembolism after total hip replacement: a randomised, double-blind, non-inferiority trial. Lancet 2007;370:949–56.

14. RE-MOBILIZE Writing Committee, Ginsberg JS, Davidson BL, Comp PC, et al. Oral thrombin inhibitor dabigatran etexilate vs North American enoxaparin regimen for prevention of venous thromboembolism after knee arthroplasty surgery. J Arthroplasty 2009;24:1–9.

15. Colwell CW, Spiro TE. Efficacy and safety of enoxaparin to prevent deep vein thrombosis after hip arthroplasty. Clin Orthop Relat Res 1995;319:215.

16. Ezekowitz MD, Reilly PA, Nehmiz G, et al. Dabigatran with or without concomitant aspirin compared with warfarin alone in patients with nonvalvular atrial fibrillation (PETRO Study). Am J Cardiol 2007;100:1419–26.

17. Connolly SJ, Ezekowitz MD, Yusuf S, et al. RE-LY Steering Committee and Investigators. Dabigatran versus warfarin in patients with atrial fibrillation. N Engl J Med. 2009;361:1139–1.

18. Kakar P, Watson T, Lip GYH. Drug evaluation: Rivaroxaban, an oral, direct inhibitor of activated Factor X. Curr Opin Investig Drugs 2007;8:256–65.

19. Kubitza D, Becka M, Wensing G, et al. Safety, pharmacodynamics, and pharmacokinetics of BAY 59-7939 – an oral, direct Factor Xa inhibitor – after multiple dosing in healthy male subjects. Eur J Clin Pharmacol 2005;61:873–80.

20. Eriksson BI, Borris LC, Dahl OE, et al. ODIXa-HIP Study Investigators. A once-daily, oral, direct Factor Xa inhibitor, rivaroxaban (BAY 59-7939), for thromboprophylaxis after total hip replacement. Circulation 2006;114:2374–81.

21. Eriksson BI, Borris L, Dahl OE, et al.; ODIXa-HIP Study Investigators. Oral, direct Factor Xa inhibition with BAY 59-7939 for the prevention of venous thromboembolism after total hip replacement. J Thromb Haemost 2006;4:121–8.

22. Eriksson BI, Borris LC, Dahl OE, et al. Dose-escalation study of rivaroxaban (BAY 59-7939) – an oral, direct Factor Xa inhibitor – for the prevention of venous thromboembolism in patients undergoing total hip replacement. Thromb Res 2007;120:685–93.

23. Turpie AG, Fisher WD, Bauer KA, et al.; OdiXa-Knee Study Group. BAY 59-7939: an oral, direct factor Xa inhibitor for the prevention of venous thromboembolism in patients after total knee replacement. A phase II dose-ranging study. J Thromb Haemost 2005;3:2479–86.

24. Fisher WD, Eriksson BI, Bauer KA, et al. Rivaroxaban for thromboprophylaxis after orthopaedic surgery: pooled analysis of two studies. Thromb Haemost 2007;97:931–7.

25. Eriksson BI, Borris LC, Friedman RJ, et al.; RECORD1 Study Group. Rivaroxaban versus enoxaparin for thromboprophylaxis after hip arthroplasty. N Engl J Med 2008;358:2765–75.

26. Lassen MR, Ageno W, Borris LC, et al.; RECORD3 Investigators. Rivaroxaban versus enoxaparin for thromboprophylaxis after total knee arthroplasty. N Engl J Med 2008;358:2776–86.

27. Kakkar AK, Brenner B, Dahl OE, et al.; RECORD2 Investigators. Extended duration rivaroxaban versus short-term enoxaparin for the prevention of venous thromboembolism after total hip arthroplasty: a double-blind, randomised controlled trial. Lancet 2008;372:31–9.

28. Turpie AG, Lassen MR, Davidson BL, et al.; RECORD4 Investigators. Rivaroxaban versus enoxaparin for thromboprophylaxis after total knee arthroplasty (RECORD4): a randomised trial. Lancet 2009;9676:1673–80.

29. Agnelli G, Gallus A, Goldhaber SZ, et al.; ODIXa-DVT Study Investigators. Treatment of proximal deep-vein thrombosis with the oral direct Factor Xa inhibitor rivaroxaban (BAY 59-7939): the ODIXa- DVT (oral direct Factor Xa inhibitor BAY 59-7939 in patients with acute symptomatic deep-vein thrombosis) study. Circulation 2007;116:180–7.

30. Buller HR, Lensing AW, Prins MH, et al.; Einstein-DVT Dose-Ranging Study investigators. A dose-ranging study evaluating once-daily oral administration of the factor Xa inhibitor rivaroxaban in the treatment of patients with acute symptomatic deep vein thrombosis. The EINSTEIN- DVT Dose-Ranging Study. Blood 2008;112:2242–7.

31. Mega JL, Braunwald E, Mohanavelu S, et al.; ATLAS ACS-TIMI 46 study group.Rivaroxaban versus placebo in patients with acute coronary syndromes (ATLAS ACS-TIMI 46): a randomised, double-blind, phase II trial. Lancet 2009;374:29-38.
32. Shantsila E, Lip GY. Apixaban, an oral, direct inhibitor of activated Factor Xa. Curr Opin Investig Drugs. 2008;9:1020–33.
33. Morishima Y, Furugohri T, Honda Y, et al. Antithrombotic properties of DU-176b, a novel orally active Factor Xa inhibitor: inhibition of both arterial and venous thrombosis, and combination effects with other antithrombotic agents. J Thromb Haemost 2005;3:abstract PO511.
34. Zafar MU, Gaztanga J, Velez M, et al. A phase-I study to assess the antithrombotic properties of DU-176b: an orally active direct Factor-Xa inhibitor. J Am Coll Cardiol 2006;47:288A.
35. Agnelli G, Haas S, Ginsberg JS, et al. A phase II study of the oral factor Xa inhibitor LY517717 for the prevention of venous thromboembolism after hip or knee replacement. J Thromb Haemost 2007;5:746–53.
36. Eriksson BI, Turpie AGG, Lassen MR, et al. YM150, an oral direct Factor Xa inhibitor, as prophylaxis for venous thromboembolism in patients with elective primary hip replacement surgery. A dose escalation study. Blood 2005;106:abstract 1865.
37. Turpie AG, Gent M, Bauer K, et al. Evaluation of the Factor Xa (FXa) inhibitor, PRT054021 (PRT021), against enoxaparin in a randomized trial for the prevention of venous thromboembolic events after total knee replacement (EXPERT). J Thromb Haemost 2007;5;abstract P-T-652.

Chapter 6

Future directions

Eduard Shantsila, Gregory YH Lip

The large number of novel oral anticoagulants under clinical development reflects the huge clinical demand for such medicines and the desire of the pharmaceutical industry to respond to the as yet unmet needs of patients. Chronic life-long prevention of thromboembolic stroke in atrial fibrillation, an increasingly common cardiac arrhythmia, represents the largest need for oral anticoagulants, and they are required by millions of patients worldwide. Improvements in the diagnosis of venous thromboembolic events such as pulmonary embolisation, along with growing appreciation of their high prevalence and life-threatening nature, have increased the demand for convenient and reliable long-term anticoagulation.

In addition to having an irreplaceable role in venous thrombosis, effectiveness of inhibitors of the coagulation cascade in clinical settings of arterial thrombosis, such as myocardial infarction and acute coronary syndromes, is being extensively evaluated. At present, antiplatelet drugs dominate in this field. However, it appears that continuous enhancement of the potency of antiplatelet agents has its own natural limits. Breaching of these limits may provide a certain amount of benefit in terms of prevention of thrombosis but it has a downside, as evidenced by the high rate of severe haemorrhage and even by the impairment of immune responses and activation of silent cancers. The process of arterial thrombosis, although initiated by the formation of predominantly platelet clots, has numerous links with coagulation factors and often includes a significant fibrin component. Consequently, parenteral anticoagulants such as heparin have become an important part of management of patients with arterial thrombosis. Not surprisingly, several novel oral anticoagulants are being tested on patients with acute coronary syndromes.

The promise of convenient long-term anticoagulation may itself lengthen the list of potential indications for novel anticoagulants. For example, patients with various chronic conditions, such as heart failure, certain cancers and prolonged immobilisation, are known to bear high risks of thrombotic complications and thus may benefit from anticoagulant therapy if it can be provided conveniently and safely.

What would be the characteristics of the ideal anticoagulant? To make it convenient for long-term use, it would be available for oral administration. The onset of full anticoagulant action would be quick and stable throughout the day (ideally with a once-daily regimen). The anticoagulant effects would be predictable with fixed doses and would not require routine laboratory monitoring. The drug would have minimal – if any – interactions with other medicines and food. And ultimately, it must have a good safety profile in terms of risks of haemorrhage and possible effects on other organs (eg, the kidney or liver).

Can such a drug be developed in the near future? Most probably, the answer will be 'yes'. Two novel oral anticoagulants, dabigatran etexilate (a direct thrombin inhibitor) and rivaroxaban (an oral factor Xa inhibitor), have already been approved for venous thromboembolism (VTE) prevention in patients after major joint surgery. These drugs largely correspond to the requirements of an ideal anticoagulant. Furthermore, as they both participate in late stages of the coagulation cascade, their inhibition allows disruption of both the intrinsic and the extrinsic pathways. From this 'double' action stems their high antithrombotic efficacy. The results of large clinical trials of these agents in VTE and of their evaluation in a wider range of indications are eagerly awaited.